Sheffield Hallam University
Learning and Information Services
Withdrawn From Stock

Sheffield Hallam University
Learning and IT Services
Collegiate Learning Centre
Collegiate Crescent Campus
She

D1326315

Spasticity Management

Spasticity Management
A Practical Multidisciplinary Guide

Edited by

Valerie L Stevenson

Consultant Neurologist
The National Hospital for Neurology and Neurosurgery
Queen Square
London

Louise Jarrett

Clinical Nurse Specialist in Spasticity Management
The National Hospital for Neurology and Neurosurgery
Queen Square
London

Foreword by Alan J Thompson

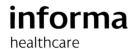
informa
healthcare

© 2006 Informa Healthcare, an imprint of Informa UK Limited

First published in the United Kingdom in 2006
by Informa Healthcare, an imprint of Informa Limited, 4 Park Square, Milton Park, Abingdon,
Oxon OX14 4RN

Tel.:   +44 (0)20 7017 6000
Fax.:   +44 (0)20 7017 6699
Website: http://www.tandf.co.uk/medicine
E-mail: info.medicine@tandf.co.uk

All rights reserved. No part of this publication may be reproduced, stored in a retrieval system,
or transmitted, in any form or by any means, electronic, mechanical, photocopying, recording,
or otherwise, without the prior permission of the publisher or in accordance with the provisions
of the Copyright, Designs and Patents Act 1988 or under the terms of any licence permitting
limited copying issued by the Copyright Licensing Agency, 90 Tottenham Court Road, London
W1P 0LP.

Although every effort has been made to ensure that all owners of copyright material have been
acknowledged in this publication, we would be glad to acknowledge in subsequent reprints or
editions any omissions brought to our attention.

Although every effort has been made to ensure that drug doses and other information are
presented accurately in this publication, the ultimate responsibility rests with the prescribing
physician. Neither the publishers nor the authors can be held responsible for errors or for any
consequences arising from the use of information contained herein. For detailed prescribing
information or instructions on the use of any product or procedure discussed herein, please
consult the prescribing information or instructional material issued by the manufacturer.

A CIP record for this book is available from the British Library.

Library of Congress Cataloging-in-Publication Data

Data available on application

ISBN 1 84184 560 4
ISBN 978 1 84184 560 9

Distributed in North and South America by

Taylor & Francis
6000 Broken Sound Parkway, NW, (Suite 300)
Boca Raton, FL 33487, USA

Within Continental USA
Tel: 800 272 7737;   Fax: 800 374 3401
Outside Continental USA
Tel: 561 994 0555;   Fax: 561 361 6018
E-mail: orders@crcpress.com

Distributed in the rest of the world by
Thomson Publishing Services
Cheriton House
North Way
Andover, Hampshire SP10 5BE, UK
Tel: +44 (0)1264 332424
E-mail: tps.tandfsalesorder@thomson.com

Composition by J&L Composition, Filey, North Yorkshire
Printed and bound in Singapore by Kyodo

Contents

Contributors

Katrina Buchanan
Clinical Specialist Physiotherapist in Spasticity
Management and Multiple Sclerosis
The National Hospital for Neurology and
Neurosurgery
Queen Square
London

Louise Jarrett
Clinical Nurse Specialist in Spasticity Management
The National Hospital for Neurology and
Neurosurgery
Queen Square
London

Louise J Lockley
Clinical Specialist Physiotherapist in Spasticity
Management and Multiple Sclerosis
The National Hospital for Neurology and
Neurosurgery
Queen Square
London

Jonathan F Marsden
MRC Clinician Scientist and Physiotherapist
Institute of Neurology
Queen Square
London

Valerie L Stevenson
Consultant Neurologist
The National Hospital for Neurology and
Neurosurgery
Queen Square
London

Foreword

Spasticity is a poorly recognised but common symptom, present in a wide range of neurological conditions. It can have a major impact on those affected, much of which is potentially preventable. However, the combination of lack of awareness, poor understanding and inadequate management often results in this symptom having a far greater impact than necessary.

In essence, *Spasticity Management: A Practical Multidisciplinary Guide* provides an excellent paradigm to incorporate many of the key elements fundamental to the management of chronic conditions. These include

- a multidisciplinary approach with the patient and carer, an integral part of the team
- broad expertise which includes physiology, neurology, nursing, physiotherapy and occupational therapy

- a comprehensive management plan ranging from the provision of information to the availability of invasive procedures when appropriate
- continuing joined-up care to manage and monitor both the spasticity and the underlying condition causing it.

This excellent text takes a practical, pragmatic and patient-focused approach to the management of spasticity. It is accessible and relevant and will undoubtedly be an invaluable guide to all practitioners involved in providing care to patients with chronic neurological conditions.

Alan J Thompson
The National Hospital for
Neurology and Neurosurgery
Queen Square
London

Preface

The impact of spasticity on an individual can be devastating. It can cause a myriad of symptoms, and each individual's experiences are different. Although spasticity is often considered a disorder of motor function, some people with spasticity will perceive pain while others will experience discomfort or stiffness, and spasms may be described as simply annoying or as extremely painful. Chronic pain or spasms frequently interfere with sleep, and can also have an emotional impact on, for example, mood, self-image or motivation.

The presence of spasticity or spasms can obviously also impact on function. With regard to mobility, walking may be slower or more difficult, falls more frequent, or the ability to self-propel a wheelchair or transfer compromised. Likewise, activities of daily living, including washing, dressing, toileting and sexual activity, can all be affected.

All of these aspects can have a detrimental affect on the ability of an individual to continue in employment or education, or impact on fulfilment of life roles, including those as a parent or partner.

Poorly managed spasticity can also have serious long-term consequences. Muscle shortening and tendon or soft tissue contracture can lead to restriction of passive movement or physical deformity. Once contractures are present, these are often very difficult to treat and can have major functional implications, including difficulties in carrying out personal hygiene or dressing. With severe contractures, positioning can be affected, resulting in an inability to seat an individual, which will inevitably lead to restricted community mobility and social isolation. In addition, through compromising positioning in sitting or lying, contractures can lead to the development of pressure sores, which may in turn increase the severity of spasticity and spasms, resulting in a vicious circle.

Awareness of these implications, early identification, and intervention to treat spasticity and associated symptoms such as spasms can minimise development of these long-term secondary complications.

Finally, it must not be forgotten that, as well as contributing to these complications and loss of function, spasticity may also be useful for an individual, perhaps allowing them to stand or walk when their weakness would not otherwise permit it.

With these issues in mind, it is imperative that management always be individualised and function focused rather than simply being aimed at the reduction of spasticity as a sign or symptom.

So, is another book on spasticity really needed? Several books and review articles dealing with spasticity have been published over recent years, so it could be argued that there is no need for another. This would indeed be the case if this book simply explained the pathophysiology of spasticity and listed its possible causes and treatments. Several excellent publications have covered this area; however, none of these is a truly practical guide relevant to all members of the multidisciplinary team involved in management of the individual with spasticity. Several of these previous publications are excellent sources of information – and are referenced here accordingly – but often the information that is needed by a multidisciplinary team faced with a particularly challenging problem or with developing a service is nowhere to be found. Anyone who has been involved in setting up a new service knows how difficult and how protracted a process this can be, so any help or guidance is usually greatly valued.

The idea for this book has been growing over the last few years and has been nurtured by visitors to our service, of all disciplines from many different National Health Service (NHS) Trusts in the UK, as well as visitors from overseas. Feedback has on the whole been very good, but the recurring theme from visitors has been the desire to take our protocols and guidelines and replicate the service elsewhere. This seems to be a good idea, but a busy NHS clinic has not proved an appropriate place to be able to impart details of our experience to others.

Consequently, the basis of this book is to collect together the experience and knowledge of a multidisciplinary team who have worked in this area for over 10 years. It draws together several areas, including basic knowledge of pathophysiology, how to set up and develop a service, as well as useful management strategies and treatment interventions. On a practical note, it includes complete copies of the patient information that we have developed and found useful, proformas for assessing individuals, protocols for different interventions, nursing care plans, and an integrated care pathway for outpatient spasticity management. These protocols are, of course, specific to our service, but could easily be adapted and tailored specifically for use in other centres.

This is not, however, an exhaustive text, and there are clearly some areas that are not covered in detail as they fall outside our area of expertise – for instance, specialist seating and orthotics, and the details of neurosurgical procedures. These areas are clearly referenced to allow easy access to more information.

We are not claiming that this is the 'right' or only way to run a spasticity service, and there is certainly room for improvement, but we hope that by sharing our experience we can help others to develop their own service and thus improve management for all individuals with spasticity.

One of the recurring themes throughout this book is the emphasis on the importance of all team members being involved in providing education to the person with spasticity and if appropriate their carers and families. We believe strongly that by facilitating individuals with spasticity to learn how to manage their own symptoms and become 'expert patients', many of the previously common consequences of suboptimally managed spasticity can be avoided. Before we can educate others, we do of course need a sound knowledge base of our own. Optimum management of spasticity is dependent on an understanding of its underlying physiology, an awareness of its natural history, an appreciation of the impact on an individual, and a comprehensive approach to minimising that impact that is both multidisciplinary and responsive over time.

Valerie L Stevenson
Louise Jarrett

Acknowledgements

The spasticity service at the National Hospital for Neurology and Neurosurgery has evolved over the last 10 years. During this time, several different professionals have worked within it, all of whom have been instrumental in its development and day to day running. Many of these individuals have also helped compile the patient information and protocols included within this book, and we are grateful to all of them. However, we would particularly like to acknowledge the following people;

- Professor Alan J Thompson for his vision to initiate the service and mentorship of the team as the service has evolved, as well as for reviewing and commenting on an earlier draft of this book
- Davina Richardson (Specialist Neuro-Physiotherapist) for her input to earlier versions of the measurement form and the spasticity and botulinum toxin information leaflets
- Bernie Porter (Consultant MS Nurse) for involvement in the development of the nurse's role in intrathecal baclofen therapy and her input into earlier versions of the medical protocol, patient information, and service development algorithm (Table 8.2)
- Michael Powell (Consultant Neurosurgeon) in his ongoing commitment to refine the surgical technique in order to prevent complications following implant of the intrathecal pumps (Appendix 11)
- Lisa Buckley (Spasticity Management Nurse Specialist) for her review and comments on earlier versions of Chapters 3 and 7 and the associated appendices, as well as for her assistance with the illustrations
- Karen Baker (Senior 1 Neuro-Physiotherapist) for her helpful comments on an earlier version of Chapter 4
- Clive Woodard (National Business Development Manager, Medtronic Neurological Division) for his review and comments on the intrathecal baclofen section of Chapter 7
- Paul Nandi (Consultant Pain Management Anaesthetist), Denise Colbeck (Pain Management Nurse Specialist), and Christine Eastman, Artemis Ghiai and Lisa Englishby (Pain Management Nurses) for their role in the development of the phenol service and for reviewing the intrathecal phenol section in Chapter 7 and its associated appendices
- Rory O'Connor (Rehabilitation Consultant) for an earlier version of Figures 7.6 and 7.8 and his input into the development phase of the integrated care pathway (Appendix 1)
- Kevin O'Hara (Technical Instructor, Therapy Services) for his assistance with the illustrations

Finally, and most importantly, we should like to thank our patients, past and present, who through their experience and feedback have helped develop our knowledge of spasticity and who continue to guide us in evolving the service.

Section I

Chapter 1

What is spasticity?

Valerie L Stevenson and Jonathan F Marsden

'Spasticity' means different things to different people. The individual with spasticity will no doubt think of it in terms of their own symptoms and how these affect them, whereas physicians and other healthcare providers often consider spasticity as a neurological impairment. When considering how best to manage a person's symptoms or reduce the impact of these on their daily life, it may seem unimportant to think about the underlying neurophysiological changes secondary to their neurological condition. However, a sound knowledge of underlying physiology is extremely important for all members of the multidisciplinary team. This knowledge will not only guide the team in devising the most appropriate management plan for an individual, but will also allow them to provide clear and relevant education to the person with spasticity, and if appropriate their families and carers. This provision of education and promotion of self-management is instrumental in the overall success of any spasticity management programme.

The muscle stiffness of spasticity, often with associated spasms, is an extremely common symptom seen in many neurological conditions, including head or spinal cord injury, stroke, cerebral palsy, and multiple sclerosis. It is also a significant feature in a number of rarer conditions, such as hereditary spastic paraparesis. Due to the diversity of causes, it is a problem faced by many people of all ages and backgrounds. Several of these disorders predominantly affect young adults or are lifelong conditions, in contrast to stroke, which is predominantly a disorder of older age. It is therefore essential that all health workers, whether based in hospitals or in the community, be equipped with a degree of understanding of spasticity and its appropriate management. Continuity of care and knowledge, particularly across the interfaces of primary and secondary care as well as community rehabilitation teams and care agencies, is invaluable.

DEFINITIONS OF SPASTICITY

The most well-known and referenced description of spasticity is the physiological definition proposed by Lance in 1980:[1]

> Spasticity is a motor disorder characterised by a velocity-dependent increase in tonic stretch reflexes (muscle tone) with exaggerated tendon jerks, resulting from hyperexcitability of the stretch reflex, as one component of the upper motor neurone syndrome.

According to this definition, it is only the increased resistance to passive movement (muscle tone) that is defined as spasticity – other features of the upper motor neurone (UMN) syndrome, such as spasms or clonus characterised by brief often repetitive episodes of muscle contraction, are excluded.

More recently, a European working group, EU-SPASM,[2] as part of a review of spasticity measurement and evaluation, looked at this discrepancy and Lance's definition of spasticity in detail. In the light of recent research, three specific areas of Lance's definition were felt to require modification:

- Velocity-dependent changes in limb stiffness during passive movement are not solely due to neural changes but are contributed to by the normal viscoelastic properties of soft tissues.[3]
- In addition to hyperexcitable stretch reflexes, activity in other pathways (afferent, supraspinal and changes in the α motor neurone) is also important in the development of spasticity.
- Spasticity cannot be exclusively considered a 'motor disorder', as afferent activity (cutaneous and proprioceptive) is also involved.

To reflect these aspects, the EU-SPASM group proposed a new definition of spasticity:[2]

Spasticity – disordered sensorimotor control, resulting from an upper motor neurone lesion, presenting as intermittent or sustained involuntary activation of muscles.

This term, although broader and consequently less specific, does now allow more aspects of the UMN syndrome to be included under the umbrella term of spasticity, such as spasms and clonus.

The UMN syndrome can be divided into so-called positive and negative aspects (Table 1.1). The positive aspects involve additional motor activity, including stiffness, spasms and clonus, while negative features include weakness, decreased postural responses and reduced dexterity. It must be remembered that these factors may occur independently of each other, but often it is the combination and inter-

action of the different aspects of the UMN syndrome (both positive and negative) with their functional consequences that make managing individuals so challenging.

Throughout this book, the term spasticity will be used to describe the increase in muscle tone resulting from the underlying neurological condition. Other features of the UMN syndrome, such as spasms or clonus, although included under the EU-SPASM definition of spasticity, will be mentioned specifically to highlight any particular issues or management strategies.

NORMAL TONE, MUSCLE CONTRACTION AND STRETCH REFLEXES

Muscle tone refers to the ongoing tension in a muscle, apparent as resistance experienced to passive movement and stretching. Muscle tone or stiffness at rest is influenced by several different factors: the passive (or non-neural) component due to viscoelastic properties of connective tissue and muscles crossing the joint, and a neural component due to the stretch reflex.[4] In healthy subjects, stretch reflexes are only elicited with high-velocity stretches (e.g. as seen with a tendon jerk); the resistance felt to slow passive movement is due solely to the viscoelastic component. In addition, when a contracting muscle is stretched, there is a further component to the resistance felt due to tension in active cross-bridges that are present within the muscle (intrinsic stiffness). Stretch reflexes, through their contribution to limb stiffness, are therefore important in helping to maintain posture and in the control of limb movement.

STRETCH REFLEXES

Skeletal muscles are innervated by lower motor neurones that originate in the ventral horns of the spinal cord. In response to muscle stretch, sensory axons arising from specialised receptors (muscle spindles) embedded within connective tissue capsules in the muscle are activated. These sensory axons (group Ia and II afferents) relay information to the brain and spinal cord from the spindles about length changes (both amplitude and speed of stretch) of the muscle. Within the ventral horn of the spinal cord, the sensory axons form monosynaptic excitatory connections

Table 1.1 Features of the upper motor neurone (UMN) syndrome

Positive	Negative
Spasticity	Weakness
Spasms	Reduced dexterity
Clonus	Reduced postural responses
Associated reactions	
Positive support reaction	
Brisk tendon reflexes	
Extensor plantar responses	

with α motor neurones supplying the same muscle, leading to a contraction of that muscle. Clinically, this can be seen as a tendon reflex such as the knee or ankle jerk and is known as a phasic (monosynaptic) stretch reflex (Figure 1.1). This pathway can be assessed experimentally by electrically stimulating Ia nerve afferents in the peripheral nerve. This activates the α motor neurones from the same muscle, and the subsequent muscle activation is measured using electrodes placed on the muscle: this is called the H reflex.[5]

Integration of muscle spindle information within the spinal cord

In addition to activating the α motor neurone as part of the stretch reflex, muscle spindle information is processed further within the spinal cord. For example, there are inhibitory connections to the α motor neurones of antagonistic muscles. Thus, as well as a rapid contraction of the stretched muscle, there is a simultaneous relaxation of the antagonist muscle – a process called reciprocal inhibition.

Figure 1.1

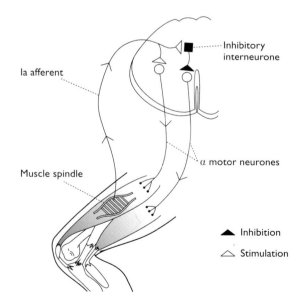

Inhibitory interneurone

Ia afferent

α motor neurones

Muscle spindle

▲ Inhibition

△ Stimulation

The monosynaptic stretch reflex and reciprocal inhibition. Adapted from: Mayer NH. Clinicophysiologic concepts of spasticity and motor dysfunction in adults with an upper motoneuron lesion. Muscle Nerve 1997; Suppl 6:S21–3. Reproduced with permission.

Modulation of the monosynaptic stretch reflex

As well as reciprocal inhibition, there are other inhibitory circuits within the spinal cord that can modulate the size of the stretch reflex, either by affecting the transmission of muscle spindle sensory information (via presynaptic inhibition) or via excitability of the α motor neurone. During the contraction of an agonist muscle, these mechanisms act to inhibit stretch reflexes within the antagonist muscle that may otherwise interfere with the movement.[6,7]

Modulation may also occur via descending pyramidal (corticospinal) or parapyramidal pathways. The pyramidal tract arises from the motor areas of the cerebral cortex, while parapyramidal pathways arise from the brainstem (in particular within the vestibular nucleus, superior colliculus and reticular formation). Signals through these pathways may activate inhibitory spinal circuits, but can also directly affect the excitability of the α motor neurone.[8] As well as these descending signals, sensory inputs from various sources (e.g. cutaneous stimuli) can also activate inhibitory spinal cord circuits and thus affect stretch reflex size.

Finally, the muscle spindle is also modulated by the activity of γ motor neurones within the spinal cord. These motor neurones innervate specialised intrafusal fibres within the muscle spindles. Activating the intrafusal fibres will alter the sensitivity of the muscle spindle and thus the size of the muscle spindle afferent response for a given stretch.

Factors affecting stretch reflex size

Reflecting the multiple mechanisms by which stretch reflexes can be modulated, there are many factors that may influence the size of the monosynaptic stretch (or H) reflex. Reflex amplitude can, for example, vary with the position of the person (e.g. supine versus sitting) and the position of the head and limbs.[5] These changes are probably mediated by alterations in the sensory input to the central nervous system.

Muscle activity in distant body parts can also affect stretch reflex size: for example, clenching the teeth can affect the size of reflexes recorded in the arm and the leg.[9–11] This finding is used clinically in the Jendrassik (reinforcement) manoeuvre, whereby distant muscle activity is used to enhance the reflexes that are being tested.

As a result of the many factors that may influence stretch reflex activity, it is important to standardise as much as possible the position and activity of the person when assessing and re-assessing tone.

Stretch reflex changes during functional movement

The size of the short-latency monosynaptic stretch reflex is also modulated by tasks such as standing. Further modulation occurs during walking, with the stretch reflex size varying throughout the different phases of walking: for example, in the calf muscles, it is higher during the stance phase than the swing phase.[12–14] Such control and modulation occur through changes in motor neuronal and spinal cord inhibitory interneuronal activity. The inhibition of the stretch reflex during the swing phase of walking may facilitate accurate foot placement. In contrast, the higher stretch reflex size during the stance phase may allow a person to rapidly correct for any irregularities in the ground as well as contributing to push off at the end of the stance phase.[15] It is clear from this example how integral stretch reflexes are to the normal control of movement.

Long-latency stretch reflexes

When a contracting muscle is stretched, there is an increase in stretch reflex amplitude. Longer-latency stretch reflexes are also seen in addition to the monosynaptic short-latency stretch reflex. The causes of these later stretch reflexes vary between different muscles. In the hand muscles, for example, sensory signals from the muscle spindle activate pyramidal cells within the motor cortex that in turn activate the muscle (a transcortical stretch reflex).[16,17] In other muscles, later stretch reflexes may be caused by signals from the slower-conducting group II afferents (rather than Ia) or via further processing through the spinal cord (oligosynaptic pathways).[18] These longer-latency stretch reflexes are very adaptable: for example, their sizes may vary considerably, depending on the degree to which the person tries to resist the forthcoming stretch.[16] This degree of cognitive influence reflects the large supraspinal control over these longer-latency reflexes and means they are very effective in altering limb stiffness so that it is appropriate to the task at hand.

Stretch reflexes and spasticity

As Lance[1] described, in spasticity there is a 'velocity-dependent increase in tonic stretch reflexes'. This velocity dependence can be appreciated clinically by the fact that at slow velocities of movement, often no or only a minimal increase in tone is detectable; however, at faster rates, an increase in tone is clearly apparent. This increase in the tone, or strength of contraction, is directly related to the velocity of the passive movement. In spasticity, the stretch-evoked muscle contraction occurs at a short latency – consistent with a monosynaptic response. However, the stretch reflex lasts for a longer period of time (a tonic stretch reflex). Interestingly, these long-lasting tonic stretch reflexes are not present in healthy subjects when they are stretched at rest, and therefore it is not clear if this is a new reflex that appears in the UMN syndrome or merely a change in the gain or threshold, which are set extremely high in healthy subjects.[19–22]

Clasp knife phenomenon

This clinical sign has been described as one of the characteristics of limb stiffness (hypertonia) secondary to spasticity. It refers to the almost sudden reduction in tone that occurs when moving a limb with spasticity. At first when the limb is moved, there is a gradual increase in resistance opposing the stretch, which then suddenly appears to release. The reasons for this clinical change are twofold. Firstly, as the resistance to movement increases, the velocity of the movement declines and the stimulus evoking a tonic stretch reflex is reduced. Secondly, tonic stretch reflexes appear to be not only velocity-dependent but also length-dependent; thus, as muscles are stretched further, the sensitivity to stretch reflexes is actually reduced. These two factors combine such that, at a certain point in a muscle stretch, the stimulus to the stretch reflex is simultaneously reduced and resistance to movement will suddenly drop.[23]

PATHOPHYSIOLOGY OF SPASTICITY

Spasticity, along with weakness, loss of fine movement, spasms, clonus and exaggerated tendon reflexes, all occur in the context of the UMN syndrome. A common misconception is that the pyramidal tracts are therefore responsible for all of these features.[23] However, lesions of this pathway or of the primary motor cortex alone may cause weakness and loss of dexterity, but do not cause the positive phenomena characteristic of the UMN syndrome, including spasticity, spasms, clonus or exaggerated reflexes. Instead, it is apparent that these features appear as a result of disruption of modulatory descending pathways. As outlined previously, the descending parapyramidal pathways, particularly the dorsal reticulospinal tract, are important in activating inhibitory spinal circuits and in controlling the threshold and rate of α motor neurone activation.[8] In keeping with this, patients with damage to these descending pathways show a decrease in spinal cord inhibitory control such as reciprocal inhibition and presynaptic inhibition.[6,7,24–27]

Although there is clearly a reduced inhibitory spinal cord control that may enhance stretch reflexes in spasticity, other factors must also be contributory. This is illustrated by two points. Firstly, a lack of spinal cord inhibitory control is also seen in other conditions, such as dystonia and Parkinson's disease,[28–31] suggesting that this is not a problem specific to people with spasticity and cannot be the sole cause of spasticity. Secondly, the slow clinical development of spasticity following a neurological insult argues against it simply being a release phenomenon with a sudden decrease of inhibitory control over the spinal cord and the onset of spasticity.[32]

Recent studies have suggested that motor neurones undergo intrinsic changes that develop over time, and it may also be possible that new pathways or connections arise over time within the spinal cord that alter how muscle spindle signals are processed. The changes in motor neurone properties result in abnormally long plateau-like potentials that prolong motor neurone discharge and thus muscle contraction in response to synaptic inputs.[33–35] Although prolonged motor neurone discharge can occur in healthy subjects, the paucity of inhibitory spinal cord control in people with spasticity means that this activity could, once triggered, continue relatively unabated. In spasticity, this may also result in a lack of reduction in stretch reflex size that is normally seen with repetitive stimulation of the muscle spindle afferents (post-activation depression).[33,36] Lesions to pathways descending from the brainstem, such as the serotonergic pathways from the raphe nucleus, may be important in driving these motor neurone changes.[37]

SPASTICITY AND FUNCTIONAL MOVEMENT

Movement always involves stretching the opposing muscle group (antagonist); in spasticity, this may elicit a stretch reflex in the antagonist muscle that is large enough to oppose the movement. For example, stretch reflexes are frequently enhanced in the finger and wrist flexors following stroke; these contribute significantly to tone[38,39] and may oppose finger and wrist extension. This is supported by the fact that botulinum toxin injections into the wrist flexors result in a significant decrease in stretch reflex activity, an increase in the range of voluntary wrist extension, and in half of the cases an improvement in hand function.[40] Similarly enhanced stretch reflexes within the lower limb plantarflexors may impair active, particularly fast, ankle dorsiflexion.[7]

As outlined earlier, when an actively contracting muscle is stretched in healthy subjects, the size of the monosynaptic stretch reflex increases. When actively contracting muscles are stretched in people with spasticity, the stretch reflex size is often similar to that seen in healthy subjects.[19,41,42] Therefore the enhanced stretch reflex activity seen at rest may not necessarily affect the person to the same degree when they are active.[41] In fact, the enhanced stretch reflex activity seen at rest in spasticity may often be because the person is unable to completely relax the muscle – this has been referred to as spastic dystonia.[23] This underlying background contraction contributes to the increase in stretch reflex size seen in people with spasticity.[42]

In contrast, other studies that have looked at stretch reflex activity during functional tasks rather than during isometric contractions have found that stretch reflexes may indeed be enhanced in spasticity when the muscle is contracted. In stroke and multiple sclerosis, for example, there is an enhanced response to a muscle stretch applied during walking, and the stretch reflexes (or H reflex) do not show a normal modulation during the swing and stance phase as described earlier.[43–46] Similarly, during natural unperturbed walking, a velocity-dependent response to calf muscle stretch is seen post stroke, which is indicative of stretch reflex hyperexcitability and spasticity. Interestingly, patients whose muscles had a greater velocity sensitivity to stretch demonstrated a slower walking speed. This suggests that stretch reflex hyperexcitability does have a negative effect on walking.[47]

The functional improvements seen with pharmacological interventions such as botulinum toxin[48] further highlight the potential importance of enhanced stretch reflexes in limiting upper and lower limb function. However, it must be remembered that studies often quantify spasticity using clinical measures such as the Ashworth score that do not distinguish between neural and non-neural contributions to tone, both of which may be affected by treatment interventions.

In conclusion, the relationship between enhanced stretch reflex activity and functional movements is complex, and a reduction in stretch reflex activity using pharmacological interventions may not always result in an improvement in the pattern of movement and function.[49] This may be because spasticity is only one component of the UMN syndrome, and other factors such as weakness and changes in passive stiffness may be as, or more, important for an individual.

OTHER FACTORS CONTRIBUTING TO STIFFNESS

Changes within the connective tissue and muscles crossing a joint can also significantly influence limb stiffness (hypertonia): this is referred to as passive, or non-neural, stiffness. In the UMN syndrome, the passive contribution to tone is often increased and develops over time following the neurological event.[45,50–52] The viscoelastic changes observed may be due to an increase in the number of attached cross-bridges in the resting muscle and/or a decrease in their detachment rate as well as changes in the intramuscular and surrounding connective tissue.[53,54] The degree of change in passive stiffness may vary across muscle groups and between individuals. Increases in passive stiffness are, for example, frequently seen in the gastrocnemius/soleus muscle complex.[45,51,52] In contrast, following stroke, passive stiffness in the long finger flexors may be normal in the presence of enhanced stretch reflex activity.[38,39] These differences may reflect variations in the amount and architecture of intramuscular connective tissue and the muscles' role in tasks such as postural control. The amount by which the muscle has been stretched will also impact on the development of non-neural changes.

Thixotropy

Muscle and connective tissue also demonstrate a phenomenon called thixotropy. This is the property whereby with repetitive movement there is a decrease in passive stiffness, similar to that seen when initially stirring a gel or a pot of paint. This means that the resistance is higher with the initial movement and decreases with subsequent movements. Although the degree of thixotropy seems similar in healthy subjects and in people with stroke, this high initial resistance may be sufficient to prevent movement in people who are very weak.[55]

The presence of thixotropy has implications for assessing tone, as resistance felt to passive movement will depend on the position and activity of the limb immediately prior to movement. Prior contraction with the muscle in a shortened position, for example, increases stiffness.[56,57] It is therefore important to take into account the impact of thixotropy when assessing tone by measuring after a predetermined and fixed number of prior movements.

Distinguishing between neural and non-neural stiffness

Connective tissue changes can occur without any contracture, and the resulting stiffness may vary in a velocity-dependent manner similar to spasticity, making it difficult to distinguish clinically between hypertonia of neural and non-neural origin.[58,59] To make this distinction is, however, clinically important, as the treatment of non-neural (passive) stiffness is via physical adjuncts such as stretching and splinting rather than pharmacological interventions. Techniques such as the Tardieu test that compare the stiffness felt with slow stretches to that felt with faster stretches may provide a clinical estimate of the passive and neural components to tone.[60–62] The slow stretch allows an assessment of the passive component in isolation, as it is slow enough not to elicit a stretch reflex, while the faster stretch elicits a stretch reflex and so the stiffness felt is a combination of the neural and non-neural components. Electromyography (EMG) is another technique that can be helpful in estimating the neural component to hypertonia, and is often used when considering botulinum toxin treatment (Chapter 6). One of the most precise ways to clinically assess the neural component to hypertonia is illustrated by the use of local anaesthetic spinal blocks in the assessment process when considering people for intrathecal phenol therapy (Chapter 7). This gives the opportunity to completely remove the neural component to stiffness, exposing solely the passive component.

It can clearly be difficult to distinguish the relative contributions of the neural and non-neural components to hypertonia. However, on a practical note, as connective tissue changes almost invariably develop in the UMN syndrome, instigating an effective stretching and moving programme is essential for all individuals, although it is not clear how much stretching is actually necessary to prevent muscle shortening (Chapter 4).

Passive stiffness and function

An increase in passive stiffness may actually have some benefits for a person, as it can compensate for an inability to actively generate muscle activity (i.e. weakness). In standing, for example, increased passive stiffness at the ankle may contribute significantly to the torque that is required at the ankle to maintain a standing posture. However, passive resistance is constantly present, unlike muscle activity, which can normally increase and decrease voluntarily. Therefore, although passive stiffness may be useful in the maintenance of posture, it may interfere with movements,[63] particularly fast ones.

Co-contraction

Abnormal co-contraction (simultaneous contraction of both agonist and antagonist muscles) can also contribute to limb stiffness. Co-contraction of muscles is of course a normal phenomenon necessary to stabilise joints and fixate position such as posture in sitting or standing, or fixing the wrist and elbow to enable a cup of tea to be carried. However, abnormal co-contraction can occur in the UMN syndrome and interferes with function by making muscles appear weaker than they are, or reducing coordination and dexterity.

Co-contraction can occur with rapid or rapidly alternating movements; in these cases, a stretch-evoked contraction of the antagonist muscle may underlie the co-contraction.[7] In other cases, co-contraction may occur without any muscle stretch or activation of the stretch reflex;[64] this may be because the normal relaxation of the antagonist muscle (via reciprocal inhibition) seen at the beginning of a contraction can change in people with spasticity to an excitatory response resulting in agonist–antagonist co-contraction.[65] Therefore the abnormalities that contribute to enhanced stretch reflexes (impaired spinal inhibitory pathways) may also contribute to the presence of co-contraction.

Detection of co-contraction is important as it has therapeutic consequences: it may be possible to pharmacologically weaken antagonist muscles, allowing agonists to work more efficiently; for example, botulinum toxin therapy to the finger flexors may allow the unopposed extensors to open the hand and grasp objects, thus returning some function to the affected hand.[66]

CLONUS

This is a rhythmic pattern of contraction occurring at a rate of several times per second and can be demonstrated by a sudden stretch of a muscle. Clonus may be a normal finding at the ankle, but is not sustainable, with usually only a few beats lasting 1–2 seconds.

In the UMN syndrome, clonus is commonly observed in the muscles of the leg, with rhythmic contractions of both the gastrocnemius and soleus muscles in response to dorsiflexion of the ankle. In individuals with soft tissue changes, simply having the feet positioned on footplates can be enough of a stretch to provoke clonus. The repetitive movement or 'jumping' is caused by the alternate stretching and unloading of the muscle spindles, which, if the stretching force is sustained, will result in continuous rhythmic triggering of the phasic stretch reflex.

SPASMS

Spasms, or sudden involuntary (often painful) movements, are frequently associated with spasticity, but physiologically their mechanism of action appears to be different to the velocity- or stretch-dependent hypertonia. Spasms may be clearly precipitated by muscle stretch, but may also be triggered via a variety of peripheral, noxious and visceral afferents, including pressure sores, bowel impaction, urinary retention or infection. Non-nociceptive cutaneous stimuli such as touch, bedclothes or tight garments may be enough to trigger spasms. So-called spontaneous spasms may well be the result of as-yet unidentified stimuli; it is therefore essential to search for any possible trigger factors, which may be cutaneous or visceral in nature. Over time, an individual's pattern of spasticity and spasms will almost invariably change and fluctuate according to the presence of trigger factors and their location.

Spasms may be predominantly flexor, extensor or a combination of both (with or without adduction). Flexor spasms (sudden ankle dorsiflexion, knee and hip flexion) can occur due to disinhibited polysynaptic reflexes such as the flexor withdrawal reflex (a normal response in humans that is triggered by a noxious stimulus to the foot such as standing on a nail) or may reflect abnormal activity within spinal cord circuits that have the effect of synchronising the discharge of motor neurones supplying multiple muscles.[67–69] Extensor spasms are triggered in much the same way as flexor spasms; whether a noxious stimulus causes flexion or extension is influenced by its location. Spasms may be so severe that both the limbs and trunk may fully extend and can cause people to fall (if walking or transferring) or compromise safety in seating systems.

ASSOCIATED REACTIONS

Individuals with UMN syndromes who are undertaking one activity with one part of the body, such as walking or using the hand for fine motor tasks, may experience involuntary activity in another part of the body. Most commonly, this is seen when a person with a hemiparesis is walking and experiences progressive flexion of the affected upper limb. The degree of associated reaction appears to be related to both the severity of hypertonia in the limb showing the associated reaction and in the effort necessary for the task.[70]

The mechanisms underlying these reactions are not clear, but probably include disturbed descending supraspinal control, perhaps through unaffected, but less focused, bulbospinal pathways taking on the role of damaged corticospinal pathways.[71]

THE POSITIVE SUPPORT REACTION

When weight bearing is achieved through a paretic leg secondary to an UMN lesion, a characteristic pattern of movement may occur, with plantarflexion and inversion of the foot with or without knee extension: this pattern of movement is known as the positive support reaction. Like flexor or extensor spasms, it is a disinhibited primitive reflex, which can be observed in the normal neonate: extension of the legs occurs on placing the feet on a hard surface and allowing a few seconds where, with support, the infant can weight-bear before the knees buckle to a

sitting position. The positive support reaction in an individual with a hemiparesis, although allowing weight bearing in an often weak leg, can unfortunately be very disabling, interfering with rehabilitation of both standing and walking as it prevents normal weight transference during the phases of walking.

CONTRACTURES

Prolonged immobility of joints and muscles in a shortened state can lead to irreversible changes in the muscles, tendons and ligaments that result in loss of passive range at joints. Within muscles, sarcomere number may be reduced and histochemical changes resembling denervation can occur.[72]

These soft tissue changes may be a consequence of increases in the neural and/or non-neural components of hypertonia, and have been noted as early as 2 months following stroke.[45,73] The presence of contractures therefore does not imply spasticity, and may be caused simply by non-neural stiffness. If weak limbs (for example as present in Guillain–Barré syndrome, an acute peripheral lower motor neurone neuropathy) are positioned incorrectly or not moved passively, contractures will occur.

Once contractures have been allowed to form, management is much more difficult and may even require surgery – prevention is therefore paramount.

SPASTICITY IN CONTEXT

The positive features of the UMN syndrome considered here are only a few of the symptoms that an individual may experience: others, such as poor balance, muscle weakness and reduced dexterity, all clearly also impact on a person's function. Accompanying the increase in the size of the short-latency monosynaptic stretch reflex characteristic of spasticity, there is often a reduction in the size of the longer-latency stretch reflexes and postural reflexes.[74–76] This is because these longer-latency reflexes are under significant cortical control, which may also be damaged by the underlying neurological event. As these longer-latency reflexes are functionally important in maintaining posture and limb stiffness appropriate to the task conditions, this loss can significantly affect balance.[74,75] Weakness may be caused by a direct lack of activity in descending pathways, resulting in abnormalities in motor unit recruitment and firing rate, as well as by secondary disuse atrophy.[77] The degree of weakness can significantly impact on function: for example, the speed of walking following stroke is directly related to the severity of lower-limb weakness.[78]

Damage to the corticospinal tract, in particular, results in poor dexterity and difficulty in performing independent fractionated finger movements. This reflects the fast, direct connections that the corticospinal tract makes to motor neurones supplying the hand muscles.[79]

Any aspects of the UMN syndrome may occur independently of another, but in reality there is often a combination of these features. It is therefore essential to carry out a detailed assessment to identify the relative contribution that each makes to an individual's reduction in function (Chapter 2). For example, in hereditary spastic paraparesis, it was often thought that spasticity was the main factor contributing to the abnormal gait, but if spasticity is effectively reduced (e.g. by intrathecal baclofen), there is often evidence of profound underlying weakness that is clearly contributing to disability.[80] This balance between weakness and spasticity is often difficult for both clinicians and people with spasticity to appreciate. It is therefore essential when considering therapeutic strategies that the goals of treatment be clearly defined and reflect the complex interactions between the symptoms and signs of the UMN syndrome while keeping the individual's level of function as the focus.

CONCLUSIONS

Having an understanding of the neurophysiological changes responsible for the clinical picture of spasticity and its associated features is essential in designing effective management plans for individuals with spasticity and their carers and families. This knowledge will enable the multidisciplinary team to select appropriate treatment interventions and to be alert to the importance of preventing long-term complications such as contractures, and will ensure that aggravating and trigger factors for spasticity and spasms are managed appropriately. With an understanding of these concepts, it will also be possible to ensure that the individual with spasticity is provided with appropriate education to arm them with the knowledge and mechanisms to monitor their own symptoms, min-

imise the development of non-neural changes and identify any trigger factors.

REFERENCES

1. Lance JW. Symposium synopsis. In: Feldman RG, Young RR, Koella WP (eds). Spasticity: Disordered Motor Control. Chicago, IL: Year Book 1980:485–94.

2. Pandyan AD, Gregoric M, Barnes MP et al. Spasticity: clinical perceptions, neurological realities and meaningful measurement. Disabil Rehabil 2005;27:2–6.

3. Dietz V. Spastic movement disorder: what is the impact of research on clinical practice? J Neurol Neurosurg Psychiatry 2003;74:820–6.

4. Sinkjaer T. Muscle, reflex and central components in the control of the ankle joint in healthy and spastic man. Acta Neurol Scand Suppl 1997;170:1–28.

5. Voerman GE, Gregoric M, Hermens HJ. Neurophysiological methods for the assessment of spasticity: the Hoffmann reflex, the tendon reflex, and the stretch reflex. Disabil Rehabil 2005;27:33–68.

6. Morita H, Crone C, Christenhuis D, Petersen NT, Nielsen JB. Modulation of presynaptic inhibition and disynaptic reciprocal Ia inhibition during voluntary movement in spasticity. Brain 2001;124:826–37.

7. Boorman GI, Lee RG, Becker WJ, Windhorst UR. Impaired 'natural reciprocal inhibition' in patients with spasticity due to incomplete spinal cord injury. Electroencephalogr Clin Neurophysiol 1996;101:84–92.

8. Brown P. Pathophysiology of spasticity. J Neurol Neurosurg Psychiatry 1994;57:773–7.

9. Boroojerdi B, Battaglia F, Muellbacher W, Cohen LG. Voluntary teeth clenching facilitates human motor system excitability. Clin Neurophysiol 2000;111:988–93.

10. Sugawara K, Kasai T. Facilitation of motor evoked potentials and H-reflexes of flexor carpi radialis muscle induced by voluntary teeth clenching. Hum Mov Sci 2002;21:203–12.

11. Miyahara T, Hagiya N, Ohyama T, Nakamura Y. Modulation of human soleus H reflex in association with voluntary clenching of the teeth. J Neurophysiol 1996;76:2033–41.

12. Zehr EP, Stein RB. What functions do reflexes serve during human locomotion? Prog Neurobiol 1999;58:185–205.

13. Sinkjaer T, Andersen JB, Larsen B. Soleus stretch reflex modulation during gait in humans. J Neurophysiol 1996;76:1112–20.

14. Capaday C, Stein RB. Amplitude modulation of the soleus H-reflex in the human during walking and standing. J Neurosci 1986;6:1308–13.

15. Dietz V. Proprioception and locomotor disorders. Nat Rev Neurosci 2002;3:781–90.

16. Matthews PB. The human stretch reflex and the motor cortex. Trends Neurosci 1991;14:87–91.

17. Palmer E, Ashby P. Evidence that a long latency stretch reflex in humans is transcortical. J Physiol 1992; 449:429–40.

18. Grey MJ, Ladouceur M, Andersen JB et al. Group II muscle afferents probably contribute to the medium latency soleus stretch reflex during walking in humans. J Physiol 2001;534:925–33.

19. Powers RK, Campbell DL, Rymer WZ. Stretch reflex dynamics in spastic elbow flexors. Ann Neurol 1989;25:32–42.

20. Thilmann AF, Fellows SJ, Ross HF. The mechanisms of spastic muscle hypertonus. Brain 1991; 114:233–44.

21. Yeo W, Ada L, O'Dwyer NJ, Neilson PD. Tonic stretch reflexes in older able-bodied people. Electromyogr Clin Neurophysiol 1998;38:273–8.

22. Sheean G. The pathophysiology of spasticity. Eur J Neurol 2002;Suppl 1:3–9.

23. Sheean G. Neurophysiology of spasticity. In: Barnes MP, Johnson GR (eds). Upper Motor Neurone Syndrome and Spasticity: Clinical Management and Neurophysiology. Cambridge: Cambridge University Press, 2001:12–78.

24. Katz R, Pierrot-Deseilligny E. Recurrent inhibition in humans. Prog Neurobiol 1999;57:325–55.

25. Crone C, Nielsen J, Petersen N et al. Disynaptic reciprocal inhibition of ankle extensors in spastic patients. Brain 1994;117:1161–8.

26. Katz R. Presynaptic inhibition in humans: a comparison between normal and spastic patients. J Physiol Paris 1999;93:379–85.

27. Stein RB. Presynaptic inhibition in humans. Prog Neurobiol 1995;47:533–44.

28. Berardelli A, Rothwell JC, Hallett M et al. The pathophysiology of primary dystonia. Brain 1998;121: 1195–212.

29. Meunier S, Pol S, Houeto JL, Vidailhet M. Abnormal reciprocal inhibition between antagonist muscles in Parkinson's disease. Brain 2000;123:1017–26.

30. Tsai CH, Chen RS, Lu CS. Reciprocal inhibition in Parkinson's disease. Acta Neurol Scand 1997;95:13–18.

31. Nakashima K, Shimoyama R, Yokoyama Y, Takahashi K. Reciprocal inhibition between the forearm muscles in patients with Parkinson's disease. Electromyogr Clin Neurophysiol 1994;34:67–72.

32. Hiersemenzel LP, Curt A, Dietz V. From spinal shock to spasticity: neuronal adaptations to a spinal cord injury. Neurology 2000;54:1574–82.

33. Aymard C, Katz R, Lafitte C et al. Presynaptic inhibition and homosynaptic depression. A comparison between lower and uppper limbs in normal human subjects and patients with hemiplegia. Brain 2000;123:1688–702.

34. Nickolls P, Collins DF, Gorman RB et al. Forces consistent with plateau-like behaviour of spinal neurons evoked in patients with spinal cord injuries. Brain 2004;127:660–70.

35. Zijdewind I, Thomas CK. Spontaneous motor unit behavior in human thenar muscles after spinal cord injury. Muscle Nerve 2001;24:952–62.

36. Schindler-Ivens S, Shields RK. Low frequency depression of H-reflexes in humans with acute and chronic spinal-cord injury. Exp Brain Res 2000; 133:233–41.

37. Bennett DJ, Li Y, Harvey PJ, Gorassini M. Evidence for plateau potentials in tail motoneurons of awake chronic spinal rats with spasticity. J Neurophysiol 2001;86:1972–82.

38. Kamper DG, Harvey RL, Suresh S, Rymer WZ. Relative contributions of neural mechanisms versus muscle mechanics in promoting finger extension deficits following stroke. Muscle Nerve 2003;28: 309–18.

39. Kamper DG, Rymer WZ. Quantitative features of the stretch response of extrinsic finger muscles in hemiparetic stroke. Muscle Nerve 2000;23:954–61.

40. Miscio G, Del Conte C, Pianca D et al. Botulinum toxin in post-stroke patients: stiffness modifications and clinical implications. J Neurol 2004;251: 189–96.

41. Ada L, Vattanasilp W, O'Dwyer NJ, Crosbie J. Does spasticity contribute to walking dysfunction after stroke? J Neurol Neurosurg Psychiatry 1998;64: 628–35.

42. Burne JA, Carleton VL, O'Dwyer NJ. The spasticity paradox: movement disorder or disorder of resting limbs? J Neurol Neurosurg Psychiatry 2005;76:47–54.

43. Sinkjaer T, Andersen JB, Nielsen JF, Hansen HJ. Soleus long-latency stretch reflexes during walking in

healthy and spastic humans. Clin Neurophysiol 1999;110:951–9.

44. Faist M, Ertel M, Berger W, Dietz V. Impaired modulation of quadriceps tendon jerk reflex during spastic gait: differences between spinal and cerebral lesions. Brain 1999;122:567–79.

45. Sinkjaer T, Andersen JB, Nielsen JF. Impaired stretch reflex and joint torque modulation during spastic gait in multiple sclerosis patients. J Neurol 1996;243: 566–74.

46. Sinkjaer T, Toft E, Hansen HJ. H-reflex modulation during gait in multiple sclerosis patients with spasticity. Acta Neurol Scand 1995;91:239–46.

47. Lamontagne A, Malouin F, Richards C. Locomotor-specific measure of spasticity of plantarflexor muscles after stroke. Arch Phys Med Rehabil 2001;82: 1696–704.

48. Francis HP, Wade DT, Turner-Stokes L et al. Does reducing spasticity translate into functional benefit? An exploratory meta-analysis. J Neurol Neurosurg Psychiatry 2004;75:1547–51.

49. Nielsen JF, Anderson JB, Sinkjaer T. Baclofen increases the soleus stretch reflex threshold in the early swing phase during walking in spastic multiple sclerosis patients. Mult Scler 2000;6:105–14.

50. Hufschmidt A, Mauritz KH. Chronic transformation of muscle in spasticity: a peripheral contribution to increased tone. J Neurol Neurosurg Psychiatry 1985; 48:676–85.

51. Toft E, Sinkjaer T, Andreassen S, Hansen HJ. Stretch responses to ankle rotation in multiple sclerosis patients with spasticity. Electroencephalogr Clin Neurophysiol 1993;89:311–18.

52. Sinkjaer T, Toft E, Larsen K et al. Non-reflex and reflex mediated ankle joint stiffness in multiple sclerosis patients with spasticity. Muscle Nerve 1993;16: 69–76.

53. Dunne JW, Singer BJ, Allison GT. Velocity dependent passive muscle stiffness. J Neurol Neurosurg Psychiatry 2003;74:283.

54. Carey JR, Burghart TP. Movement dysfunction following central nervous system lesions: a problem of neurological or muscular impairment? Phys Ther 1993;73:538–47.

55. Vattanasilp W, Ada L, Crosbie J. Contribution of thixotropy, spasticity, and contracture to ankle stiffness after stroke. J Neurol Neurosurg Psychiatry 2000;69: 34–9.

56. Hagbarth KE, Hagglund JV, Nordin M, Wallin EU. Thixotropic behaviour of human finger flexor muscles with accompanying changes in spindle and reflex responses to stretch. J Physiol 1985;368:323–42.

57. Axelson HW, Hagbarth KE. Human motor compensations for thixotropy-dependent changes in resting wrist joint position after large joint movements. Acta Physiol Scand 2003;179:389–98.

58. Dietz V. Spastic movement disorder: What is the impact of research on clinical practice? J Neurol Neurosurg Psychiatry 2003;74:820–1.

59. Singer BJ, Dunne JW, Singer KP, Allison GT. Velocity dependent passive plantarflexor resistive torque in patients with acquired brain injury. Clin Biomech 2003;18:157–65.

60. Tardieu G, Shentoub S, Delarue R. A la recherché d'une technique de mesure de la spasticite imprime avec le periodique. Rev Neurol 1954; 91:143–4.

61. Mehrholz J, Wagner K, Meissner D et al. Reliability of the Modified Tardieu Scale and the Modified Ashworth Scale in adult patients with severe brain injury: a comparison study. Clin Rehabil 2005;19: 751–9.

62. Mackey AH, Walt SE, Lobb G, Stott NS. Intraobserver reliability of the modified Tardieu scale in the upper limb of children with hemiplegia. Dev Med Child Neurol 2004;46:267–72.

63. Fitzpatrick RC. More pulsating movement. J Physiol (Lond) 2003;551:4.

64. Dewald JPA, Pope PS, Given JD et al. Abnormal muscle coactivation patterns during isometric torque generation at the elbow and shoulder in hemiparetic subjects. Brain 1995;118:495–510.

65. Crone C, Johnsen LL, Biering-Sørensen F, Nielsen JB. Appearance of reciprocal facilitation of ankle extensors from ankle flexors in patients with stroke or spinal cord injury. Brain 2003;126:495–507.

66. Brashear A, Gordon MF, Elovic E et al. Intramuscular injection of botulinum toxin for the treatment of wrist and finger spasticity after a stroke. N Engl J Med 2002;347:395–400.

67. Norton JA, Marsden JF, Day BL. Spinally generated electromyographic oscillations and spasms in a low-thoracic complete paraplegic. Mov Disord 2003; 18:101–6.

68. Schmit BD, Benz EN, Rymer WZ. Reflex mechanisms for motor impairment in spinal cord injury. Adv Exp Med Bio 2002;508:315–23.

69. Parise M, Garcia-Larrea L, Mertens P et al. Clinical use of polysynaptic flexion reflexes in the

management of spasticity with intrathecal baclofen. Electroencephalogr Clin Neurophysiol 1997;105: 141–8.

70. Dickstein R, Heffes Y, Abulaffio N. Electromyographic and positional changes in the elbows of spastic hemiparetic patients during walking. Electroenceph Clin Neurophysiol 1996;101:491–6.

71. Dewald JPA, Rymer WZ. Factors underlying abnormal posture and movement in spastic hemiparesis. In: Thilmann AF, Burke DJ, Rymer WZ (eds). Spasticity: Mechanisms and Management. Berlin: Springer-Verlag, 1993:123–38.

72. Dietz V, Ketelsen UP, Berger W, Quintern J. Motor unit involvement in spastic paresis. Relationship between leg muscle activation and histochemistry. J Neurol Sci 1986;75:89–103.

73. Malouin F, Bonneau C, Pichard L, Corriveau D. Non-reflex mediated changes in plantarflexor muscles early after stroke. Scand J Rehabil Med 1997;29:147–53.

74. Dietz V, Berger W. Interlimb coordination of posture in patients with spastic paresis. Impaired function of spinal reflexes. Brain 1984;107:965–78.

75. Nardone A, Galante M, Lucas B, Schieppati M. Stance control is not affected by paresis and reflex hyperexcitability: the case of spastic patients. J Neurol Neurosurg Psychiatry 2001;70:635–43.

76. Sinkjaer T, Andersen JB, Nielsen JF, Hansen HJ. Soleus long-latency stretch reflexes during walking in healthy and spastic humans. Clin Neurophysiol 1999;110:951–9.

77. Zijdewind I, Thomas CK. Motor unit firing during and after voluntary contractions of human thenar muscles weakened by spinal cord injury. J Neurophysiol 2003;89:2065–71.

78. Hsu AL, Tang PF, Jan MH. Analysis of impairments influencing gait velocity and asymmetry of hemiplegic patients after mild to moderate stroke. Arch Phys Med Rehabil 2003;84:1185–93.

79. Lemon RN. The G. L. Brown Prize Lecture. Cortical control of the primate hand. Exp Physiol 1993;78: 263–301.

80. Richardson D, Thompson AJ. Management of spasticity in hereditary spastic paraplegia. Physiother Res Int 1999;4:68–76.

Chapter 2

Assessment of the individual with spasticity

Valerie L Stevenson, Louise J Lockley and Louise Jarrett

Accurate assessment is the starting point to implementation of an appropriate and successful management plan for the individual with spasticity. As well as recording physical changes such as resistance to movement, weakness and contractures, the process of building up a picture of how spasticity impacts on an individual's daily life – both positively and negatively – is vitally important. Depending on the nature of the individual's neurological condition, they may also have other symptoms, and although these may not be directly related to spasticity, it is important to understand their impact on the person, as they may influence the assessment process or the selection of treatment options.

Tailoring treatment strategies to suit each individual requires detailed ongoing liaison between the person with spasticity, any carers or family members and their treating teams.[1] It is therefore important that this process of assessment begin as early as possible, preferably at the time of referral, with information gathered before the individual actually attends clinic. It will then continue during the clinic visit and following their appointment or admission via communication with the person and their referring teams.

The use of outcome measures quantitatively informs the assessment process, but should always be used in conjunction with an individualised assessment of all aspects of the person's life. The outcome measures described in this chapter are used routinely in the clinical setting and have been found to be quick and easy to use. They also provide a vital objective record that can inform future therapeutic decisions for that individual as well as assessing the efficacy of interventions in the research or audit setting.

There are of course many other quantitative measures in use in both clinical and research arenas that may be of benefit to specific individuals with spasticity. These have been extensively reviewed elsewhere.[2,3]

HOW TO PERFORM AN ASSESSMENT

Before considering how to perform the assessment, it is necessary to decide who should be doing it. Ideally, this process can become a joint exercise between the person with spasticity and the multidisciplinary team rather than separate assessments with each professional. The benefits of working as a team include the following:

- The expertise of each professional is combined in one setting to give maximum benefit to the person with spasticity at any one time.
- The person does not have to wait for referrals to other services or professionals, giving seamless and timely care.
- The team can share knowledge and experience and discuss the best way forward, with the patient being fully involved in the process.
- The experience and skills of a team assist in a person making a fully informed decision as to whether an invasive procedure (e.g. intrathecal baclofen or phenol or botulinum toxin injections) would be acceptable and beneficial to them.

- Team members can extend their knowledge and skills by working closely with other disciplines.

Individual professional assessment and interventions also have a role – particularly if more detail in one area is needed than can be given in a clinic setting or if spasticity is not severe (in which case physiotherapy assessment and treatment may be all that is required). However, regardless of the degree of spasticity or who is performing the assessment, provision of education to the individual about spasticity and in self-management strategies is essential (Chapter 3).

In more complex spasticity, the person will almost always benefit from the expertise of a team, particularly when decisions regarding invasive treatments are needed. The make-up of a spasticity team depends on the needs of the local population and how the service fits in with other health and social care providers in the area (Chapter 8). Key members of a team will probably include a physiotherapist, doctor and nurse. However, it may be that an occupational therapist bringing skills in seating, positioning, splinting and movement in activities of daily living would be advantageous with a particular client group. Close liaison is of course necessary with other professions, including continence advisors, district nurses, orthotists, wheelchair services, social care providers or any other health or social care professional who works with the individual.

The assessment process can be thought of as having two main phases: firstly the history, or what the person with spasticity can tell us about their difficulties, and secondly the examination. The examination phase can also be divided into several stages: observation (including posture, alignment and the presence of spontaneous spasms), active movement (including range and muscle strength) and resistance to passive movement (including assessing full range of movement and identifying any contractures). During these phases, observing the interaction between the person and their family or carers, including tone of voice or any emotions, can also be very informative about the degree of impact that the spasticity is having not only on the person but also on the family unit as a whole.

The history – or what the person with spasticity can tell us

The importance of taking a thorough accurate history as part of the assessment process cannot be overemphasised. Before any form of physical examination is undertaken, it is essential to engage with the person with spasticity and find out about their lifestyle and how spasticity may be impacting on this. The person's own account and expectations or hopes are crucial and will guide the direction and focus of the rest of the assessment.

It is often useful to begin with very open questions that not only guide the assessor to areas of specific concerns but can also reveal the expectations of the individual. For example:

'The purpose of this clinic appointment is to see if we can help you with any problems you are experiencing due to stiffness, spasms or difficulty moving. Are there any particular issues that concern you, or that you would like help with?'

Answers to questions such as these may vary from specific problems such as painful spasms disturbing sleep or difficulty self-catheterising due to adductor spasms that can be immediately focused on, to other wider issues such as wanting to walk again. These open questions are also a useful way to set the scene, and often allow a systematic assessment to follow naturally.

As well as allowing the person with spasticity to guide the direction of the assessment to areas that particularly concern them, it is also important to ensure that several key areas are addressed. Often these seem irrelevant to the individual, so it is important, for example, to highlight, in a sensitive manner, the link between bladder or bowel dysfunction aggravating spasticity and spasms. To ensure that these specific areas are assessed appropriately and not neglected, it is often useful to use a checklist during the assessment. An example of such a guide useful for all professionals can be found in the assessment section of the integrated care pathway (ICP) (Appendix 1). It is not anticipated that this format should be rigidly followed, as the person's account will guide the history taking and each assessment will be individualised; however, it is a useful tool to ensure that relevant areas are not missed. In our clinic, as the person discusses their main issues and how the spasticity is affecting their life, notes are made in the relevant sections of the ICP without the need for direct questioning unless further clarification is needed. This allows for a more natural flow of dialogue between the person and the team.

One useful way to ensure the impact of spasticity on an individual's life is accurately reflected is to go through a typical 24-hour day with the person and, if appropriate, their carers or family members. This will then serve as a guide for the rest of the assessment.

Questions and areas to be considered will be:

- How do they get out of bed and transfer or mobilise? Do they have any difficulties with washing or dressing due to spasticity or spasms?
- Specific tasks – for example, how do they manage car transfers, work, domestic or leisure activities?
- Is maintaining their posture and positioning throughout the day problematic? Do they manage to change position throughout the day? Is any positioning equipment utilised; if so, is it useful?
- Is sleep affected? If so, what position do they sleep in? Are they able to change position independently? What type of mattress do they have, and are any aids used for positioning? Is sleep disturbed by other factors such as bladder needs, pain or discomfort?

It is then useful to find out more about any symptoms of spasticity and what, if any, therapies have been tried:

- Establish the presence of any stiffness, spasms or pain and document their evolution. Be sure that your understanding of the terminology used is what the person is intending to describe. For instance, the words 'spasm' or 'stiffness' may be used by people to describe their feeling of neuropathic pain or perhaps weak, heavy legs. If spasms and stiffness are present, which is more problematic? If spasms are a particular concern, determine any aggravating factors such as specific movements or positions, trigger factors, or wearing off of medication. Ask specifically about the common trigger factors for spasticity or spasms:
  - *Bladder*: establish current management, history of infections, residuals, incontinence or self-regulating fluid restriction.
  - *Bowels*: establish current management, history of constipation, diarrhoea or incontinence.
  - *Skin*: are there areas of redness or vulnerable or broken pressure areas? Establish if the person can pressure-relieve and change position independently. What is the extent of any sensory deficit?
  - *Maintenance of hygiene and general health*: consider the presence of other potentially relevant conditions (e.g. ingrown toenails, deep vein thrombosis, tight-fitting clothes, splints or orthoses).
  - *Other sources of infection*: e.g. chest.
- If pain is described then determine whether this is associated with spasms or spasticity, or is due to other causes such as neuropathic or musculoskeletal factors.
- Document current medication used to manage spasticity, recording doses, route, times taken, effect and how long it lasts. Also carefully document any medication tried in the past, including the dose and schedule, any beneficial or unwanted effects, and why previous medication was discontinued.
- Are seating services involved? When was the seating last reviewed, and has the spasticity changed since then? Are postures and positions adopted during movement and at rest contributing to the spasticity, spasms or skin breakdown?
- Is a home exercise programme established? If so, what exercises are used, who prescribed them, how often are they performed, is the programme helpful and when was it last reviewed? If lower-limb spasticity is problematic and standing or walking is difficult, has a standing programme been tried?
- What is the therapy input to date. Has the person ever seen a physiotherapist or occupational therapist? If so, who, how often, and does it help the spasticity or spasms?
- Are any orthotics or splints used? If so, do they impact on the spasticity and do they cause any skin problems?
- Establish the person's knowledge about spasticity and tone management and any other useful management strategies that they incorporate into their daily life.
- Consider the impact of mood, self-image and motivation.

While the assessment is ongoing, it is useful to keep a couple of specific questions in mind:

- Is their spasticity helpful to function?
- Is the spasticity a focal or more generalised problem?

Both of these issues are important when it comes to planning therapeutic interventions.

The examination – or 'Hands On' assessment

This part of the assessment process is used to confirm the picture already described by the historical account, as well as providing an opportunity for quantitative measurement. The additional information available through a physical assessment will help guide the team in producing a tailored management programme that will reflect the relative balance between increased tone, muscle weakness and biomechanical factors, with the ultimate aim of improving function, relieving symptoms and preventing future problems. The examination can be divided into three key stages: observation, assessment of active movement and underlying muscle weakness, and assessment of resistance to passive movement.

Observation

Record posture, pattern of spasticity or spasms, presence of spontaneous spasms, seating if applicable, and patterns of movement when mobilising (e.g. walking, transferring or picking up objects). A simple written description can be invaluable when recording posture, positioning and movement patterns. Time allowing, photographs or video recordings can be useful for the team and the person to monitor the effect of interventions over time. Other measures may include the 10-metre timed walk and goniometry at rest (see the outcome measures form: Appendix 2). The extent of any pressure sores or skin changes can be recorded by photographs or by a simple measure of the area (e.g. 5 mm × 10 mm).

Assessment of active movement and underlying muscle weakness

This is useful in establishing if weakness or spasticity is the main factor limiting function or causing symptoms such as heaviness or stiffness. The relative contributions of these will clearly impact on proposed management plans. The Medical Research Council (MRC) grading scale (Table 2.1) is a universally recognised tool that is quick to use and routinely forms part of the standard neurological examination, although it is more difficult to apply when moderate or marked spasticity is present. Muscles are graded on a six-point ordinal scale, although grade 4 (active movement against gravity and resistance) can be

subdivided into 4−, 4 and 4+ according to whether resistance is mild, moderate or strong.

It may also be relevant to record the active range of movement at a joint using a simple goniometer (a long-armed protractor).

Assessment of resistance to passive movement

This is done in the limbs and trunk; any spasms elicited are also recorded. The Ashworth scale (Table 2.2) is the most widely used assessment tool to measure resistance to limb movement in a clinic setting, although it is unable to distinguish between the neural and non-neural components of increased tone.[4] The scale has been criticised mainly due to potential problems with inter-rater reliability and poor responsiveness in clinical trials.[5] However, variations in the interpretation of the degree of increased tone can be minimised by using a standard assessment technique (Table 2.3) and through consistency of examiner. The same technique should be followed by all members of the assessment team to aid in reliability of outcome measures recorded over time; recommendations can be included in an outcome measures form (Appendix 2). Despite the known deficiencies of the Ashworth scale, it remains an important clinical tool and if

Table 2.1 Medical Research Council (MRC) grading of muscle strength

Grade	Definition
0	No contraction
1	Flicker of contraction only
2	Active movement with gravity eliminated
3	Active movement against gravity
4	Active movement against gravity and resistance
5	Normal power

Table 2.2 Ashworth scale

0	No increase in muscle tone
1	Slight increase in tone giving a catch when the limb is moved
2	More marked increase in tone but limb easily moved
3	Considerable increase in tone – passive movement difficult
4	Limb is rigid in flexion or extension

Table 2.3 Recommendations to standardise the measurement of the Ashworth scale

- Perform three passive movements only and record the score of the resistance felt on the third movement
- The score is taken within the available range
- Move the limbs in the best alignment possible, record position and use when repeating measures
- Regulate the speed by counting 1001, 1002, 1003

assessed in a standardised fashion can be meaningful, especially when used to assess the effectiveness of an intervention that can make significant changes to spasticity, such as intrathecal therapies.

Estimating the contribution of the neural (neurophysiological) and non-neural (biomechanical) components of spasticity is difficult but important, as interventions will differ depending on the cause. Slowing the speed of the passive movement to minimise activation of the hyperexcitable reflexes and holding the muscle in a lengthened position (which may dampen the reflex response) has been described as useful in determining the non-neural component.[6] The Tardieu scale[7,8] considers both the velocity of movement of the limb as well as the angle at which assessment occurs (the point of minimal stretch of the muscle). By assessing resistance to limb movement at different velocities, it can help distinguish between neural and non-neural components of hypertonicity in the clinical setting. Clearly, due to the repeated measurements at specific limb angles at different velocities, it is more time-consuming to carry out than the Ashworth scale.

It is worth noting that all of the recognised spasticity scales are for limb assessment only and do not measure truncal spasticity. However, if the individual's main problem is caused by increased truncal tone and/or spasms then appropriate quantitative and qualitative assessment should be attempted to capture and reflect this. Simple verbal or visual analogue scales for truncal spasm or stiffness can be useful, but creative means of measurement may also be employed – for example, measuring the degree of active or passive trunk flexion by recording the distance between two fixed points on the trunk with a tape measure at rest and after movement.

The accurate documentation of any restrictions to passive movement caused by contractures is extremely important. Goniometry is a quick and simple method of recording the degree of contracture, and can be used at any joint.[9] Many people with spasticity will be unable to achieve the standard positions recommended for goniometry, particularly in a busy clinic setting; however, it can still be useful in any other position, provided that the specific position adopted is recorded and is used consistently throughout any subsequent measurements.

See the outcome measures form in Appendix 2.

When to assess

Assessment of an individual's spasticity can be completed during a single session; however, as spasticity is often variable over time and can change in its nature and severity throughout the day and night, often a better assessment is gained at more than one sitting. In building up a complete picture, input from other people involved in the individual's care (e.g. family members, carers or other health professionals) is often invaluable. Obtaining a true picture of a person's spasticity during the physical stage of assessment in outpatients is fraught with difficulty, as often they may have had a long journey to reach the clinic or may have taken their medication at a different time to normal. By taking a careful history and listening to all involved in the person's care, however, an accurate assessment can usually be made.

OUTCOME MEASURES

Measurement is a necessary part of the spasticity assessment. For clinicians, it can be the start of understanding what a person's spasticity feels like, it forms a quantifiable judgement, and, together with other parts of the assessment, the ways in which the spasticity affects the person's lifestyle can start to be appreciated. This can be particularly important when trying to assess how a treatment may be incorporated effectively into an individual's lifestyle or in assessing the impact of a therapeutic intervention.

Much has been written and quantitatively researched regarding this area, and many different objective measurement techniques have been employed, including clinical, biomechanical and neurophysiological methods.[2,10,11] Most of these techniques have been designed and explored in the research setting and have not as yet found their way into routine clinical practice. Despite this, they remain extremely important both in furthering our knowledge of spasticity and as tools for clinical trials.

Concern has been raised over the lack of correlation between measurement techniques involving clinical, biomechanical and neurophysiological methods;[10] however, this simply highlights the fact that measures from different domains may complement each other by representing different aspects of spasticity and its impact.[12]

The choice of clinical scales to reflect the degree of spasticity and its impact on the individual is extensive, although most available scales[2] are single-item measures with poor reliability, validity and responsiveness.[12] To try to address these problems, a new scale has been developed in the multiple sclerosis (MS) population (The Multiple Sclerosis Society Spasticity Scale, MSSS-88). This is an 88-item, patient-based, interval-level scale that not only looks at spasticity symptoms but also incorporates the person's experience of spasticity and how spasticity affects their daily life.[12] The MSSS-88 scale has yet to be evaluated in people with spasticity due to conditions other than MS, but appears to have great potential as a further measurement tool to complement existing biomechanical and neurophysiological techniques.

In clinical practice, when selecting outcome measures, there clearly needs to be a balance between ease and speed of use and validity, reliability and responsiveness. Unfortunately, many of the available objective measures developed within the research arena are time-consuming to employ and require expensive equipment. In addition, the person being measured often has to be able to adopt a standardised posture – something that is often impossible for people with significant disabilities to do both physically and comfortably. It is therefore clear that selection of appropriate outcome measures for use within the clinical setting depends not only on defining exactly what is important to measure but also on practicality of use. A selection of different measures is probably most appropriate to reflect the different aspects of the condition.[3]

The limited use of objective measures in everyday clinical assessment of spasticity probably reflects the time available and the varied nature of spasticity, as well as the often complex nature of the patients. However, on a practical note, in our everyday practice, we have found a few simple scales with minimal equipment (essentially just a goniometer and tape measure) to be extremely useful. We routinely use a battery of measures to reflect different aspects of spasticity, such as range of active and passive movement, resistance to passive movement, muscle strength, and clonus and spasm frequency, as well as subjective measures to capture the individual's perspective, such as VAS (visual or verbal analogue scale) for pain, stiffness and comfort over 24 hours. In addition, relevant functional measures (e.g. timed walks, the nine-hole peg test and speech comprehension scores) may be included. The exact battery of scores used is individualised for each patient to reflect their particular problems. For any intrathecal trials or treatment with botulinum toxin, the most important tool is the negotiated goal, which is related to the person's main problem. The success of an intervention can be assessed by whether or not this goal is achieved.

The outcome measures form in Appendix 2 was developed as a measurement tool for people admitted to the National Hospital for Neurology and Neurosurgery (NHNN), London with moderate to severe spasticity for further assessment or for trials of intrathecal baclofen or phenol; with this in mind, it concentrates on lower limb spasticity and its consequences. The form contains measures that we have found clinically relevant and easy to perform in an inpatient setting, with a combination of both health professional- and patient-rated scores. The measures are used in the context of our general comprehensive assessment to guide treatment and reflect the outcome of any intervention. They do not replace but rather complement the holistic assessment, and are intended to inform decision making with the individual and the team.

The majority of the measures are evidence-based and consequently referenced, but due to the lack of suitable measures to reflect some aspects of spasticity and the effects that spasticity can have on a person's life, there are a few non-evidence-based scores included that we as a team have found useful in clinical practice. The measures that we routinely use are as follows:

- *Goniometry.* This essentially uses a long-armed hinged protractor that measures the angle at a joint by aligning each arm with the limb or trunk.[9] Measures can be performed at any joint, but are commonly recorded at the hip, knee and ankle when assessing individuals for potential intrathecal therapies. Guidance for positioning during measurement is included in the outcome measures form (Appendix 2); however, if the person being measured finds these positions uncomfortable, any posture can be adopted, provided that this is recorded and the same position is used during future assessments. Measurements are always recorded for the resting angle and full passive range. Additional recordings can be made for the active range if appropriate.

- *Range of passive hip abduction.* This is simply the maximum distance between the knees measured using a tape measure when the hips are passively abducted with the patient in the supine position.[13] If an alternative position is used, this should be recorded.
- *Ashworth scale.* This is an ordinal scale of tone intensity with five grades from 0 to 4 (Table 2.2). Although it is the most well-known and used scale, reliability may be problematic, particularly with regard to inter-rater variability.[4,5]
- *Adductor tone rating.* This is a further five-point ordinal rating of tone, but is confined to the adductors.[14]
- *Spasm frequency scale.* This is an ordinal rank scale (0–4) based on self-reporting of lower-limb spasm frequency in people with spinal cord-related spasticity. It is scored depending on how many spasms are experienced in an average hour.[15]
- *Clonus and spasms score (self-report).* This is a further ordinal scale (0–3), based on self-reporting of the frequency and provocation of both spasms and clonus.[16]
- *Numeric rating pain intensity scale (NRS).* This is a verbal analogue scale that asks the person to rate their pain on a scale of 0–10.[17]
- *Numeric rating scale for leg stiffness.* This is a verbal analogue scale that asks the person to rate their level of stiffness on a scale of 0–10.
- *Posture in seating score.* This is a self-designed score comprising four simple yes/no answers that are assigned scores of 1/0 and when summed give an estimate of seating posture (score of 0–4). In addition, baseline sitting tolerance is estimated and scored 1–4 according to tolerance levels of more than 6 hours, reducing to less than 1 hour.
- *Walking and falls score.* This is an estimate of fall frequency scored in an ordinal fashion (0–4), with 0 being no falls and 4 equating to more than 1 per day. If appropriate, a timed 10-metre walk is also recorded.[18]

- *Overall comfort rating.* This is a verbal analogue scale that asks the person to rate their level of comfort over the preceding 24-hour period on a scale of 0–10. This has been included in addition to the pain NRS following an observation by the team that regularly pre-treatment, people recorded no pain but after treatment stated they felt more comfortable.

Goal setting

The fundamental question that we need to ask ourselves as clinicians is why are we treating the spasticity? More importantly, the person with spasticity wants to know what the treatment or intervention is likely to achieve. Whether an intervention or treatment is perceived as successful will depend totally on what the aims of treatment are. A therapy that reduces the Ashworth scale from 3 to 2 in the legs but makes no difference to a difficult transfer may on paper look effective to clinicians but to the individual receiving the treatment be considered worthless.

In order to evaluate if interventions are effective, a goal of treatment needs to be set with the individual and if appropriate their carers or family. This goal is an invaluable and quantifiable measuring tool that is completely focused on the individual and their personal priorities. It does, however, have to be realistic, and it is important that if the person has unrealistic hopes or expectations of a treatment, such as being able to walk again, then these are carefully and sensitively explored. Although it is often appropriate to maintain some hope, colluding with unachievable aims must be avoided. Often with the involvement of family or carers, it is usually possible to agree a goal that will make a difference to the person's life but is also achievable. The goal agreed will be completely individualised to each person and should focus on what will actually make a difference to his or her life, not to changes visible during a treatment session or stay in hospital.

Spasticity is complex and affects people in many different ways and in all areas of their lives. To easily quantify the effects of an intervention, it may be best to focus on one specific goal, for example:

- to sit safely in the wheelchair
- to be able to sleep through the night
- for my carer to be able to do intermittent catheterisation more easily

- for my carer to be able to clean my left hand
- to be able to walk more comfortably

The emphasis on goal-setting keeps the individual and the team focused on the most important issue and also acts as a monitor for successful therapy over time by ensuring the initial goal achievement is maintained.

Outcome measures, audit and research

The documentation of the agreed goal and battery of measures is clearly helpful in the assessment of an individual and in guiding management decisions. However, routine collection of data on the whole population referred to the service or receiving a particular intervention can also be useful to guide appropriate service developments that reflect the specific client population, or in assessing the efficacy or side-effects of therapeutic interventions.

Other clinical governance issues are also important, including risk management: if invasive treatments such as intrathecal baclofen or phenol are carried out, it is extremely useful to have clear documentation of the decision-making process, including objective measures obtained before and after trials of therapies. These measures are also invaluable in managing expectations of therapeutic interventions and can be used to guide consent processes.

BEING MEASURED – PERSPECTIVES FROM PEOPLE WITH SPASTICITY

The area that is generally neglected when discussing and researching the use of outcome measures is the impact that being measured has on the person.

What is it like for the person with spasticity to be measured? Often these people have severe complex disabilities, which they are managing as best they can and have been doing so for a significant period of time. Some people successfully merge their disability into their daily lives and it does not dominate, whereas for other people their symptoms and underlying impairments can be a focus of how they choose to lead their lives.[19] Issues around self-image and confidence, or how people wish to be perceived by others, can be compounded by measurement of their spasticity. The nature of measurement means that as health professionals, we try to quantify what we see and make a valued judgement both subjectively and objectively. This can trigger people to focus on how their body is changing, which can be a threat to how they have envisaged or constructed themselves within the context of their illness.[20,21] When we measure, we concentrate on the detail of how much we can move limbs and how they feel when we do so. We also ask the individual to focus on what their main problem is and what would be the one thing that could improve their current lifestyle. Measurement is often recorded as numbers and verbally shared between 'measurers', for example stating Ashworth scores or ranges of movement as the limb is moved – frequently these have little or no meaning to the person with spasticity.

In our clinical practice, people have responded to the measurement process both positively and negatively.

Positive statements include the following:

'It feels really good to be stretched like this, it hasn't happened for years'
'It is really good that someone is taking such an interest in my spasticity'

On the other hand, we can also get negative statements, such as the following:

'Is it good or bad?'
'Have I passed the test? Will I be able to get a pump now?'

Being measured can make people feel as if they are being tested or judged. Healthcare professionals need to be aware of these issues and use strategies to minimise these feelings in individuals when carrying out measurements. Ensuring that the measurement process is not a threatening process can be achieved by paying attention to several key areas:

- Provision of education to people with spasticity about why measurement is required, how it will help the assessment and what their role in it is.
- Emphasising to the individual that being measured is not a test and there are no right or wrong results – that it is simply a way of helping the team to understand their spasticity and therefore consider potential treatments and advise on how these may impact on the person's daily life.

- Actively engaging the person in the measurement process. This may require creativity and flexibility, particularly in those individuals with a significant degree of cognitive impairment. It may involve engaging with individuals when they are most able, for example at particular times of the day, or breaking the assessment into small sections to ensure they do not fatigue. Otherwise, it may be important to have the close involvement of a significant other or main carer who could add to the overall assessment by providing a perspective on how the outcome may affect the person's lifestyle and care routine at home.

- Utilising measurement tools that involve self-reporting, such as visual and verbal analogue scales. These can help the person or carer to feel part of the process. They also often encourage the individual to focus and to be able to be more specific about the changes that they feel in their bodies. They can help the family to perceive changes in the person's body and the ways in which these may impact at home; this is particularly important during therapeutic trials of intrathecal drugs.

- Expert practitioners have been described as being able to 'reflect in the moment' – analysing the reactions of those around them and taking appropriate action as they practise.[22] The act of actually looking back or reflecting on a situation in real time has been questioned, and the idea has been developed of expert practitioners being 'mindful as they practise'.[23] This is more than being aware and taking action – it involves being actively alert to cues that may mean that a person is not coping, or is finding a situation difficult. Such cues will have been identified through pattern recognition while working over time with people having similar experiences; expertise is developed through acknowledging these patterns and working with the individual to address them.[24] The negative quotes above would be classed as cues that would make the expert practitioner stop and address these issues with the individual. So, another key intervention could be suggested as the practitioner being 'mindful when measuring'.

USING THE ASSESSMENT AND OUTCOME MEASUREMENT INFORMATION TO FORMULATE A MANAGEMENT PLAN

Several algorithms have been devised over the years to guide the management of spasticity; however, these all rely on careful and accurate assessment.[25–27] These algorithms are clearly not suited to all clinical settings or teams, but they are useful models that can be adapted to particular work environments. In our clinical setting, we have found it useful to develop an algorithm to guide the teams within the hospital when confronted with problematic spasticity; this can be initiated on first contact and assessment, prior to involving the specialist spasticity team (Figure 2.1).

However, not every health provision setting or team finds the use of algorithms useful in promoting thoughtful and comprehensive management schemes. An alternative way of looking at the provision of timely intervention is to consider the impact and severity of spasticity on a continuum from mild to severe (Table 2.4). By assessing an individual's spasticity and the impact it has on their life, the likely management needs can then be seen.[27]

CONCLUSIONS

Comprehensive and accurate assessment of an individual's spasticity and related symptoms and the effects that these have on their life and of those around them is essential in the development and implementation of an appropriate and successful management plan for that individual. Incorporating some simple outcome measures into this process provides a mechanism to record changes over time and the effects of any therapeutic intervention. It is essential that the person with spasticity feel comfortable and involved in this process and that the main goal of therapy be realistic, relevant and beneficial to them and their lifestyle.

Figure 2.1

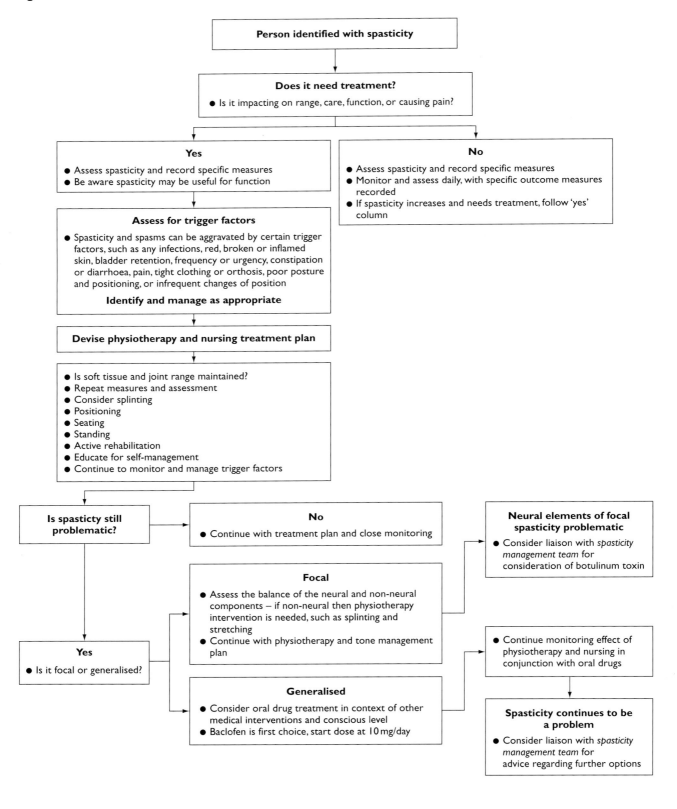

Algorithm for inpatient spasticity management at the National Hospital for Neurology and Neurosurgery, London

Table 2.4 The severity, impact and potential management options of spasticity[a]

Mild spasticity

- Clonus or mild increase in tone

- No or minimal loss of range

- Mild spasms; generally not problematic, or impacting on function, but annoying or inconvenient

Emphasis on self-management, education, and how to seek help to prevent secondary complications.

- Highlight potential trigger factors

- Education of secondary complications

- Stretches: neurophysiotherapist identifies vulnerable areas and recommends specific, active and regular stretches

- Discuss ways of maintaining active movement and modify patterns of movement to minimise increasing spasticity

- Low-dose medication targeted at problematic times of the day, with ongoing review and evaluation, may be beneficial

Moderate spasticity

- Loss of range of movement and possible contracture

- Walking is often effortful, and may require aid or wheelchair

- Difficulty releasing grip or in hand hygiene

- Minor adaptations required for position in lying: T-roll, wedge, pillows, lumbar roll

Emphasis on early identification and treatment of trigger factors, review of self-management knowledge, and liaison with team members involved throughout the different healthcare sectors. Maximise the use of oral drugs and consider the use of botulinum toxin if focal.

- Identify trigger factors and treat as appropriate

- Targeted neurophysiotherapy; active stretching, exercise and standing programmes, consider splinting

- Maximise available activity to positively impact on function and establish extent spasticity and spasms are used to enable effective movement, consider rehabilitation

- Accurately document assessments and treatments to enable ongoing evaluation of intervention

- Maximise oral drugs and consider whether botulinum toxin could be helpful for focal spasticity

- Consider referral to specialist service

Severe spasticity

- Marked increase in tone

- Loss of range and probable contracture

- Often hoisted for transfers

- Difficult positioning despite complex seating systems

- Reduced skin integrity

- Often reliant on a catheter and regular enemas

Emphasis on maximising use of oral and focal drug treatments while considering use of intrathecal baclofen or phenol. Review individuals, carers and health team management strategies.

- Identify trigger factors and treat as appropriate

- Accurately document assessments and treatments to enable ongoing evaluation of intervention

- Assess effectiveness of current treatment strategies, modify as appropriate and consider intrathecal drugs

- If intrathecal drugs are used, review need to reassess seating, transfers and therapy input. Consider rehabilitation

- If treatments are or become ineffective, review management strategies, including possibility of surgery

[a] Adapted with permission from: Thompson AJ, Jarrett L, Lockley L et al. Clinical management of spasticity. J Neurol Neurosurg Psychiatry 2005;76;459–63.

REFERENCES

1. Jarrett L. The role of the nurse in the management of spasticity. Nurs Residential Care 2004;6:116–19.

2. Platz T, Eickhof C, Nuyens G, Vuadens P. Clinical scales for the assessment of spasticity, associated phenomena, and function: a systematic review of the literature. Disabil Rehabil 2005;27:7–18.

3. Burridge JH, Wood DE, Hermens HJ et al. Theoretical and methodological considerations in the measurement of spasticity. Disabil Rehabil 2005;27:69–80.

4. Ashworth B. Preliminary trial of carisoprodal in multiple sclerosis. Practitioner 1964;192:540–2.

5. Hass BM, Bergstrom E, Jamous A, Bennie A. The inter rater reliability of the original and of the modified Ashworth scale for the assessment of spasticity in patients with spinal cord injury. Spinal Cord 1996;34:560–4.

6. Boyd RN, Ada L. Physiotherapy management of spasticity. In: Barnes MP, Johnson GR (eds). Upper Motor Neurone Syndrome and Spasticity: Clinical Management and Neurophysiology. Cambridge: Cambridge University Press, 2001:96–121.

7. Tardieu G, Shentoub S, Delarue R. A la recherché d'une technique de mesure de la spasticite imprime avec le periodique. Rev Neurol 1954;91:143–4.

8. Boyd RN, Graham HK. Objective measurement of clinical findings in the use of botulinum toxin A in the management of children with cerebral palsy. Eur J Neurol 1999;6(Suppl 4):S23–35.

9. Norkin CC, White DJ. Measurement of Joint Motion: A Guide to Goniometry. Philadelphia, PA: FA Davis, 1985.

10. Wood DE, Burridge JH, Van Wijck FM et al. Biomechanical approaches applied to the lower and upper limb for the measurement of spasticity: a systematic review of the literature. Disabil Rehabil 2005;27:19–32.

11. Voerman GE, Gregoric M, Hermens HJ. Neurophysiological methods for the assessment of spasticity: the Hoffmann reflex, the tendon reflex, and the stretch reflex. Disabil Rehabil 2005;27:33–68.

12. Hobart J, Riazi A, Thompson A et al. Getting the measure of spasticity in MS: The Multiple Sclerosis Society Spasticity Scale (MSSS-88). Brain 2006;129(Pt1):224–34.

13. Hyman N, Barnes M, Bhakta B et al. Botulinum toxin (Dysport) treatment of hip adductor spasticity in multiple sclerosis: a prospective, randomised, double blind, placebo controlled, dose ranging study. J Neurol Neurosurg Psychiatry 2000;68:707–12.

14. Snow BJ, Tsui JKC, Bhatt MH et al. Treatment of spasticity with botulinum toxin: a double blind study. Ann Neurol 1990;28:512–15.

15. Penn RD, Savoy SM, Corcos D et al. Intrathecal baclofen for severe spinal spasticity. N Engl J Med 1989;320:1517–21.

16. Smith C, Birnbaum G, Carlter JL et al. Tizanidine treatment of spasticity caused by multiple sclerosis: results of a double-blind, placebo-controlled trial. US Tizanidine Study Group. Neurology 1994;44:S34–42.

17. Kremer E, Atkinson JH, Ignelzi RJ. Measurement of pain: patient preference does not confound pain measurement. Pain 1981;10:241–8.

18. Wade DT, Wood VA, Heller A et al. Walking after stroke: measurement and recovery over the first three months. Scand J Rehabil Med 1987;19:25–30.

19. Jarrett L, Johns C. Constructing a reflexive narrative. In: Johns C, Freshwater D (eds). Transforming Nursing through Reflective Practice, 2nd edn. Oxford: Blackwell, 2005:162–79.

20. Charmaz K. Loss of self: A fundamental form of suffering in the chronically ill. Sociol Health Illness 1983;5:168–95.

21. Kralik D. The quest for ordinariness: transition experienced by midlife woman living with chronic illness. J Adv Nurs 2002;39:1146–54.

22. Schon D. Educating the Reflective Practitioner. San Francisco, CA: Jossey-Bass, 1987.

23. Johns C. Becoming a Reflective Practitioner, 2nd edn. Oxford: Blackwell Science, 2004.

24. Benner P, Tanner C, Chelsa C. Expertise in Nursing Practice. New York: Springer-Verlag, 1996.

25. Barnes MP. An overview of the clinical management of spasticity. In: Barnes MP, Johnson GR (eds). Upper Motor Neurone Syndrome and Spasticity: Clinical Management and Neurophysiology. Cambridge: Cambridge University Press, 2001:1–11.

26. Ward AB. A summary of spasticity management – a treatment algorithm. Eur J Neurol 2002;9(Suppl 1): 48–52.

27. Thompson AJ, Jarrett L, Lockley L et al. Clinical management of spasticity. J Neurol Neurosurg Psychiatry 2005;76:459–63.

Chapter 3

Provision of education and promoting self-management

Louise Jarrett

Historically, patients have received a paternalistic style of management in the UK National Health Service (NHS), being on the receiving end of treatments or interventions rather than forming an active partnership with health and social care professionals over decisions about their care. It is now recognised that quality of care and outcomes of interventions can be enhanced by individuals having an increased understanding of their own conditions. This has led to the development of self-management courses known as Expert Patient Programmes.[1] Putting the patient as the focus of health and social care service delivery remains at the forefront of the UK Government's agenda[2,3] and is emphasised in the National Service Framework (NSF) for long-term conditions.[4] The first of the 11 quality requirements of the NSF, 'A person-centred service', states the need for health services to provide individuals with effective and timely information, education about their condition, while also involving them in decisions about their treatment and future plan of care.

This chapter aims to outline how involvement of the person with spasticity, their family or carers is central to the overall success of managing spasticity. The first part of the chapter will outline the impact of spasticity on the person, the need for active multi-disciplinary teamwork and communication across health and social care sectors, and how the success of management is dependent on effective, timely education of the person and, if appropriate, their carers.

The second part of the chapter will discuss a foundation level of knowledge to consider teaching people with spasticity and will detail the content and rationale for sections included in a patient information leaflet on spasticity management (Appendix 3). Further patient information leaflets that we have developed in conjunction with users of our service are referenced throughout the relevant chapters and are also included in the appendices: exercise (Appendix 4), botulinum toxin (Appendix 5), intrathecal baclofen therapy (Appendix 6) and intrathecal phenol therapy (Appendix 7).

THE IMPACT OF SPASTICITY

Before considering how to promote self-management through education, it is vital to have a clear idea of the impact of spasticity on an individual and what their understanding of it is. As each person's experience is so different, there is no uniform management plan – which makes managing an individual's spasticity so challenging. Reasons why management is so complex have been alluded to in Chapter 1, but it is useful to reconsider how people with spasticity may describe their feeling and experience of spasticity and spasms. With spasticity, they may describe their affected limbs or trunk as stiff or difficult to move and often associated with a 'pulling' or 'tugging' pain or discomfort. Some can define the feeling of stiffness and weakness, while others find distinguishing between the two words and what they feel difficult; likewise, some may use the word 'heavy', but this may relate to either weakness or stiffness. This confusion with terminology between health professionals and patients is important and should always be clarified to avoid misinterpretation of symptoms. If spasms are present, they can be described as aggravating, tiring or embarrassing, and can also cause discomfort or pain. All of these symptoms can impact on a person's ability to carry out aspects of daily activities such as sleeping, walking, transferring, washing and dressing. Similarly, spasticity and spasms can also affect people emotionally – for example by altering their mood, self-image or motivation.[5–7] Poorly managed spasticity can unfortunately result in muscle shortening and the development of tendon and soft tissue contractures. Once present, these are often very difficult to treat and can have major functional implications, particularly in maintaining personal hygiene and positioning.[8] Contractures may also lead to compromised safety when the person is sitting or lying and to the development of pressure sores, which in turn may increase the severity of spasms and spasticity.[9] However, it is important to remember that spasticity is not always detrimental; some people are able to stand, walk or transfer through relying on their lower-limb spasticity.[8]

The occurrence of spasticity and its associated symptoms can span the trajectory of an individual's neurological condition, and its management tends to be ongoing over time; for some, this will be a significant amount of their lifetime. The person's care is often managed by several different disciplines across health and social care sectors, all of which are responsible for offering their support to enable the individual to incorporate management and treatment strategies into their daily life. As input is from several sources and not from one team or service in isolation, coordination of management and provision of education and services across health and social care sectors is essential.

THE ROLE OF THE PERSON WITH SPASTICITY IN HIS OR HER OWN MANAGEMENT

The majority of the work associated with managing any long-term condition is done in the individual's home and community, with a small fraction of it occurring in the hospital environment.[10,11] Predominantly, the person with spasticity carries out this work, supported and (for some) assisted by their family. Encouragement, support and advice to maintain this balance, as well as periodic treatment or intervention by professionals across health and social care sectors, can enable the individual to successfully incorporate management techniques into their daily life. At certain points along this trajectory, management strategies may falter and an individual may require specialist input, perhaps with invasive treatments that require hospital admission (Figure 3.1).

The key to successful spasticity management is to ensure that such interventions are completed in an effective and timely fashion – a process that is dependent on excellent verbal and written communication

Figure 3.1

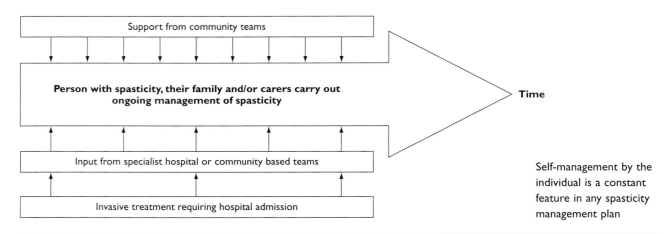

Self-management by the individual is a constant feature in any spasticity management plan

Figure 3.2

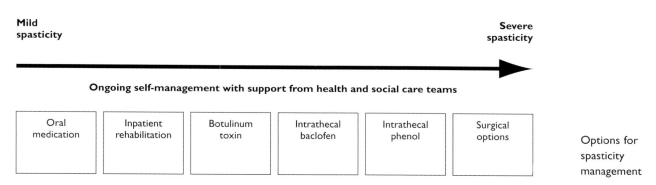

with agreed goals and integration of seamless team-work across health and social care sectors, involving the person with spasticity and their carers at all stages. Such continuity of care and documentation of the evolving impact of spasticity enables ongoing assessment of change and the appropriate choice and timing of any management intervention. Linking care pathways across healthcare sectors has been identified in recent government publications as one way to promote continuity of quality care.[4,12,13]

Involving the individual in decision-making

Treatments to manage spasticity can be considered on a continuum from mild to severe spasticity (Figure 3.2), with a constant feature of maintenance work being done by the individual and/or their care team (see the section below: 'What does the person with spasticity need to know?'). However, in reality, the timing and selection of these treatments do not follow such a linear pattern, and it is not uncommon for different treatments to be used in conjunction with each other; Figure 3.3 gives a more realistic representation of this. For example, a person using intrathecal baclofen to manage their lower-limb spasticity may also require a focal botulinum toxin injection to treat increased spasticity of their elbow flexors (a detailed discussion of the various treatments available can be found in subsequent chapters).

This concept of using different treatments at the same time can appear very confusing for the individual unless they, and their carers and families, are fully involved in the decision-making processes. The provision of appropriate education to the individual throughout this time can help to reduce anxiety about whether there are any other treatment options available or what these entail. It also guides the individual

in making informed decisions about whether such treatments or interventions are for them.

INCORPORATING EDUCATION OF THE PERSON WITH SPASTICITY INTO THE MANAGEMENT PROCESS

For spasticity management plans to be successful, the person with spasticity clearly needs to be central to the process, ensuring that the main aim or goal of treatment is appropriate and beneficial to their needs. To maximise the involvement of the individual, their education must become an integral part of the management process. The individual and their family may

Figure 3.3

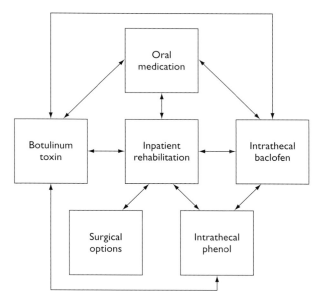

Spasticity treatments are often used in conjunction with each other

benefit from knowing about the neurological condition, its associated features and what affects them, and how they can help manage and prevent symptoms or secondary complications.[8] The timing of education provision is often said to be important,[14] but the practice of this is frequently left to the discretion and experience of the professional. An outline of a typical spasticity assessment and management process is given in Table 3.1, where key issues to consider and points of education for each stage are suggested.

Providing verbal and written information

There are many different aspects to consider when delivering education to patients, family members and/or carers (Table 3.2). Some of these are obvious, such as allowing enough time and providing appropriate written literature to back up verbal discussions,[14] but others require more thought, as each individual is different and may have specific needs – for instance an individual's level of cognitive function may need to be taken into account when preparing and giving information.

Table 3.2 outlines some of the more usual issues to consider, including tips for producing clearly written medical information suggested by the Crystal Mark Plain English Campaign.[15]

What does the person with spasticity need to know?

As with the fact that teams cannot work in isolation to manage spasticity, any single treatment cannot independently manage spasticity. There is always the need for ongoing effective general management, which is essential to optimise other treatment strategies and prevent secondary complications such as contractures. Essentially, this work focuses on maintaining movement, adequate positioning and preventing factors that may aggravate or trigger spasticity and spasms. The individual with spasticity and their carers are key to this process by ensuring that such strategies are incorporated into normal daily life.

Maintaining movement and adequate positioning

Of paramount importance in any spasticity management plan is regular movement of muscles and joints through their available range, either by the person with spasticity or passively by another person.

Maintaining muscle length can also be achieved through stretching regimes, including standing or splinting.[8] In addition, regular review of a person's lying and sitting postures and whether equipment is required to optimise these positions will facilitate the maintenance of muscle length and range of movement (Chapter 4).

Very often, the involvement of specialist and complex seating experts is essential to provide the necessary expertise to manage a person's posture over time. Their skill at the timing and provision of different seating systems throughout the person's disease course cannot be overestimated. When considering invasive treatments that will radically alter a person's posture, such as intrathecal phenol (Chapter 7), it is prudent to engage in dialogue with the relevant specialist seating service early, so that the timing of the treatment can coincide with any seating changes that may be required.

While these interventions are important and perhaps even obvious to the professional, for the person with spasticity the thought of, for example, incorporating exercises, stretches or a T-roll when sleeping into their daily routine can be daunting, a hindrance, effortful or just plain boring. This is compounded by the fact that often any changes are subtle and perhaps are more to do with maintaining function and preventing complications rather than necessarily improving the person's current situation.

When providing education and suggestions about these issues, the professional needs to be sensitive to the person's lifestyle and what level of support they have and realistic about what can be achieved and incorporated into the person's daily life. Finding time for these things can be a huge challenge for individuals who may also be busy working and being a partner, parent or friend. For instance, one woman realised that in her hectic lifestyle of maintaining a home for her husband and two children, the one thing she made time for regularly was watching her favourite television programme. She planned to use that 30-minute slot, three times a week to coincide with using her standing frame. Jointly working out with an individual how they can incorporate an exercise programme into their routine activities may be as helpful to the person as verbalising and providing written information on the importance of exercise. These issues are discussed in more detail with an example of a patient information leaflet on exercise in Chapter 4 and Appendix 4.

Table 3.1   Integrating the management and education process

Steps in the management process	Key issues for the professional to consider	Points of education and involvement for the person with spasticity
1. Accurate assessment and measurement (Chapter 2)	• Listen to the person with spasticity and their family and carers. What are the main problems? • Seek information from other teams. What do they think the main problems are? What interventions have they tried? What promoted or prevented the interventions from being successful?	• Why an assessment is needed • What they may expect in the assessment • What their role is in the assessment • What the roles are of different team members • Why measures are needed, what they may expect and what their role is during measurement
2. Feedback findings of assessment. Discuss any potential treatment options	• What do the individual and their carers and family understand about their neurological condition, spasticity or associated symptoms? • Ensure that all information is in a format understandable to the individual; consider providing written as well as verbal information	• Causes and pathology of their condition or symptoms • Details of the proposed treatment, including side-effects • Written information about the condition, symptoms and overview of potential treatments • Provide a contact number for further information
3. Establish and agree a goal of intervention	• This needs to be from the person's perspective, not the professionals' • The goal needs to affect the person's daily lifestyle, not just during a treatment session or their time in hospital • Be clear with your responses, not vague or open to misinterpretation • Be honest if the goals that the person suggests are unrealistic. Aim to maintain some hope, but not to collude with unachievable aims	• Encourage them to participate and voice their views • Provide written information outlining the goal
Communicate the goal and plan to all involved in the individual's care	• This facilitates active communication, teamwork and coordinated care so that each team member can work towards the same endpoint	• Ensure that the individual has copies of all communications in an appropriate format
4. Clearly plan the steps toward the goal and agree a plan of intervention	• A defined pathway allows the person to judge whether they want to embark upon it and participate in the work or not • Include time for assimilation of facts and for them to ask questions during and after the session • Consider timeframes, but try to be flexible to accommodate the length of time that may be required for individuals to learn about treatments and consider whether they wish to go ahead	• It is important that they take enough time to assimilate the facts and consider all the options before deciding to proceed • Review previous written or verbal information, with time for questions • It may be useful to discuss potential treatments with family members or carers

Table 3.1   continued

Steps in the management process	Key issues for the professional to consider	Points of education and involvement for the person with spasticity
5. Establish who is best placed to provide the planned interventions, to monitor their effectiveness, to provide education to the individual and to assess whether the goal is achieved	• This may require different professionals or teams at different stages. For instance, a specialist team may recommend a change in oral drugs, the GP would prescribe them and the individual (with support from their district nurse) would titrate the dose, while the community physiotherapist would help the individual to monitor the effect on their spasticity and spasms • Potential outcomes and side-effects of treatments need to be communicated to all involved • A coordinated approach across primary and secondary care may negate the need for individuals to attend many different appointments • Consider supplementary material to verbal education, including written information, website addresses, charity contact details, self-help groups or auditory recorded information	• Details of the treatment proposed, including side-effects and which healthcare professional will support them at each stage • Consider how other aspects of their health may be affected if a hospital admission or community session is required. Give details of the planned treatments and their role in them, and provide an estimate of their duration • Provide a contact number for further information from both hospital and community teams • Ensure that emergency contact procedures are communicated clearly both verbally and in writing
6. Formulate feedback strategies to all involved in the person's care so that deviations from the planned route can be assessed and reviewed, or, if the intervention is successful, so that this episode of treatment can be closed	• Effective feedback allows heathcare professionals to learn and develop their skills	• Consider the most acceptable form of feedback for the person with spasticity to use (e.g. telephone, carer or family contact)

Recognising and preventing factors that may exacerbate spasticity and spasms

The other important way to minimise spasticity and spasms is to limit unwanted sensory stimuli. Cutaneous or visceral stimuli (Table 3.3) send impulses to the spinal cord that are normally regulated by interneuronal activity. However, if these modulatory pathways are compromised, polysynaptic reflexes such as the flexor withdrawal reflex (a normal response in humans that is triggered by a noxious stimulus to the foot such as standing on a nail) can be

disinhibited, causing spasms (Chapter 1). Similarly, abnormal activity within spinal cord circuits may have the effect of synchronising the discharge of motor neurones supplying multiple muscles and thus exacerbate spasticity.[16–18]

Many people with spasticity may have recognised a link between, for example, their bowel function and spasms, but may not be aware of how actively managing such issues can impact on their overall well-being. Prevention and appropriate management of these stimuli are vital to successful spasticity treatment.

Table 3.2   Issues to consider when providing education

Verbal education

- Does the environment provide enough privacy?

- Would the person benefit from a family member or carer being involved in the education session?

- Have you got time to give adequate information? If not, can you give a brief overall summary, provide written information, and arrange another time to discuss the issues in more detail either in person or over the telephone?

- Do you need any equipment to illustrate the discussion, such as a prototype intrathecal pump or photographs of a pump refill?

- Remain aware that the individual may fatigue or need the education session broken down into smaller sections or repeated to enable understanding of the issues

- Structuring the discussion around written information provides consistency and can help to reduce anxiety at reading new material

- Ensure that the service provides a mechanism to answer any further questions that a person may have after an initial discussion. Provide contact details to allow this

Written information

- Is the information written clearly and succinctly? Use everyday words and short sentences of 15–20 words. Longer sentences should not contain more than three pieces of information. Use mainly 'active' verbs, not 'passive' ones. Avoid jargon or abbreviations

- A question-and-answer format can be helpful

- Is it in a font (12 or greater), appropriate language and format that the person can read and understand? If not, can you change it, or provide an audio or translated copy?

- Would a glossary help?

- Would pictures or diagrams increase clarity?

- In text, write numbers one to nine as words, with 10 and upwards as figures. However, be flexible: e.g. with medicines it is clearer to write 'Take 2 tablets 4 times a day'

- Use lower-case bold for emphasis, not block capitals, and avoid underlining

- Put complex information into bullet points

- Include the authors' names, date of publication and contact numbers for further information

Table 3.3   Cutaneous and visceral stimuli that may aggravate spasticity or spasms

Cutaneous stimuli	*Visceral stimuli*

- Altered skin integrity:
  – Red or inflamed skin
  – Broken skin
  – Infected skin
  – Pressure sores
  – Ingrown toenails
- Tight-fitting clothes or urinary leg bag straps
- Uncomfortable orthotics or seating systems
	- Any systemic or localised infection
	- Bowel dysfunction: e.g. constipation, overflow or diarrhoea
	- Bladder dysfunction: e.g. infections, retention or incomplete emptying
	- Deep-vein thrombosis

Key education points for people with spasticity include the following:

- *Optimisation of bladder and bowel management.* Any change such as urinary retention or infection, constipation or diarrhoea can exacerbate spasticity. Even mild infections (e.g. *Candida*) can lead to a marked increase in spasticity and spasms.
- *Maintaining skin integrity.* Preventing skin irritation, breakdown, infection and pressure sores minimises the risk of triggering spasticity. Paying close attention to maintaining hygiene not only promotes healthy skin but can also identify and monitor areas of skin at risk, for example by observing any reddening or marking from tight-fitting clothes or orthoses. Other spasticity trigger factors such as ingrown toenails or deep-vein thrombosis can also be prevented or identified at an early stage.

Understanding the significance of and effectively managing trigger factors are paramount in the management of spasticity, irrespective of other treatment options used. If a person complains of increasing spasticity or related symptoms, it is important to check for the presence of any trigger factors and start treating them before instigating new spasticity treatment regimes or changing existing ones. For instance, some women notice a change in their level of spasticity during menstruation; this may only last a few days, and simply needs understanding and explaining without the need to change medication or management strategies.

However, sometimes changes in treatments may be required until the trigger has been successfully treated and the person can then return to their original drug prescription and treatment regime; for example, a woman experienced an increase in spasticity and flexor spasms after dislocating her little toe. She had an open wound on the side of her toe and was unable to stand in her standing frame for 2 months. During this time, her partner instigated passive lower-limb stretches once a day and her intrathecal baclofen dose was increased until the bone and wound were healed and she could resume standing again. To promote her safety, she was also reminded that the increased intrathecal baclofen dose could impact on her trunk stability and hence the effectiveness of her sliding board transfers. The spasticity team regularly reviewed her during this period.

DEVELOPING A SPASTICITY MANAGEMENT INFORMATION LEAFLET

There is clearly a wealth of information from which the individual with spasticity can benefit to help maximise the effects of any treatment or intervention. The provision of a written information sheet to complement verbal discussions with the team has in our experience proved very useful (Appendix 3). The three main aims when developing this were:

1. To unravel the terminology associated with spasticity
2. To highlight what the person with spasticity can do to help manage their symptoms
3. To provide an overview of treatments.

Unravelling the terminology

It is useful to include a glossary or descriptions not only of spasticity but also of related terms such as spasms and clonus. This is felt necessary as people can sometimes use terms to describe their symptoms that they have heard in other contexts, yet their meaning to the clinician is different to what the person is experiencing and explaining. For instance, exploring closely with one woman the nature of her 'spasm' resulted in the team realising that she was experiencing episodic periods of neuropathic pain and not spasms; this enabled her drug treatment to be altered to specifically target the problem she was experiencing.

The leaflet (Appendix 3) also highlights that spasticity and weakness can coexist. This is an important issue to discuss with people, yet it is a complex one to understand. With severe spasticity, weakness is often harder for the person to isolate, as to them the stiffness is the dominant feature. Yet, if drug treatments are to be commenced and titrated to minimise the spasticity, any weakness may become more evident or unmasked; so this education is clearly vital. The person needs to be encouraged to feedback if a change in their spasticity exposes underlying weakness, as this could lead to a compromise of function. For instance, preserving a standing toilet transfer first thing in the morning may be crucial to the functioning of the person, so they may choose to take their drugs after this transfer has been completed. Failure to prepare people for the likelihood of exposing weakness once the spasticity is reduced can lead to incorrect conclusions that they have had an adverse reaction to the drug; some will even stop taking it, when in fact it has served its purpose of reducing spasticity. Careful titration to a lower dose may, however, enable the drug to be an effective component of that individual's management programme.

Comprehension by the individual of these issues can enable them to monitor the effect of the drugs on diminishing their spasticity, exposing their weakness and what effect this may have on their daily function. If the individual is unable to perform the monitoring, a carer and/or a health professional such as a community physiotherapist or district nurse could carry out this role. Feedback to the doctor with ongoing prescribing responsibility is essential to ensure that the effectiveness of the drug prescription continues to be monitored over time.

A further ambiguity in terminology can arise when a person describes the feeling of excessive weakness as stiffness. Often, very weak legs can feel 'heavy' and difficult to move for the individual even passively, and they can call this feeling 'stiffness'. The need for careful evaluation of the person's description and a physical examination of how the legs feel to passive movement is imperative to ensure that what is being described is the symptom being experienced. The danger of not doing so is that someone with heavy weak legs could be given an increased dose of their anti-spasticity drug that leads to further weakness, which could compromise their function and (if excessive) their trunk and upper body strength and in severe cases potentially their respiratory muscle support for breathing.

Highlighting what the person with spasticity can do

Descriptions of trigger factors are included in the information leaflet, as these are fundamental in the overall management of spasticity irrespective of the drug treatments used: the person with spasticity or their main carer are often best placed to monitor the occurrence and effect of these.

The importance of exercise, stretches and positioning in sitting or lying are also emphasised, with practical tips on how to modify spasms or clonus.

Some people develop an acute awareness of when their spasms and spasticity may be triggered: if this is the case then sometimes management plans can be adapted accordingly. For instance, some people with

multiple sclerosis report seasonal variations in their spasticity: in the warmer summer months, they may be less affected by spasticity and spasms compared with the cooler winter months, when they may need additional medication to manage their symptoms.

Provide an overview of treatments

This section provides an outline of the potential treatments available. This is included so that individuals can get an overall idea of what can be offered and what may or may not suit them. The dose ranges, common side-effects of the oral drugs and issues such as when regular liver function blood tests are recommended are included so that the individual can self-monitor that they are taking the correct doses and having the necessary follow-up. Brief descriptions of the more invasive treatments (botulinum toxin, intrathecal baclofen and phenol) are provided on this information sheet, but if these treatments are pursued then further specific education and detailed leaflets are provided (these are discussed and presented in subsequent chapters and the appendices).

CONCLUSION

Successful spasticity management plans not only rely on effective integrated teamwork with good communication, but also most importantly necessitate a focus on self-management by the person with spasticity. Appropriate ongoing education is essential to allow the individual to take an active role in maintaining function and monitoring the efficacy of any interventions, which are paramount in the provision of high-quality care. Such education must be provided in a timely fashion using appropriately prepared teaching aids such as written information sheets.

REFERENCES

1. Department of Health. The Expert Patient: A New Approach to Chronic Disease Management for the 21st Century. London: The Stationary Office, 2001.

2. Department of Health. The NHS Plan. London: The Stationary Office, 2000.

3. Department of Health. The NHS Improvement Plan – Putting People at the Heart of Public Services. London: DoH, 2004.

4. Department of Health. National Service Framework for Long-Term Conditions. London: DoH, 2005.

5. Ward N. Spasticity in multiple sclerosis. J Community Nurs 1999;13:4–10.

6. Porter B. Nursing management of spasticity. Primary Health Care 2001;11:25–9.

7. Currie R. Spasticity: a common symptom of multiple sclerosis. Nurs Stand 2001;15:47–52.

8. Thompson AJ, Jarrett L, Lockley L et al. Clinical management of spasticity. J Neurol Neurosurg Psychiatry 2005;76:459–63.

9. Jarrett L. The role of the nurse in the management of spasticity. Nurs Residential Care 2004;6:116–19.

10. Charmaz K. Loss of self: a fundamental form of suffering in the chronically ill. Sociol Health Illness 1983;5:68–195.

11. Strauss A, Corbin JM. Shaping a New Health Care System. San Francisco, CA: Jossey-Bass, 1988.

12. Department of Health. Self Care – A Real Choice. London: DoH, 2005.

13. Department of Health. Supporting People with Long Term Conditions. An NHS and Social Care Model to support local innovation and integration. London: DoH, 2005.

14. Nicklin J. Improving the quality of written information for patients. Nurs Stand 2002;16:39–44.

15. Crystal Mark Plain English Campaign. http://www.plainenglish.co.uk.

16. Schmit BD, Benz EN, Rymer WZ. Reflex mechanisms for motor impairment in spinal cord injury. Adv Exp Med Biol 2002;508:315–23.

17. Norton JA, Marsden JF, Day BL. Spinally generated electromyographic oscillations and spasms in a low-thoracic complete paraplegic. Mov Disord 2003;18:101–6.

18. Sheean G. Neurophysiology of spasticity. In: Barnes M, Johnson G (eds). Upper Motor Neurone Syndrome and Spasticity, Clinical Management and Neurophysiology. Cambridge: Cambridge University Press, 2001:12–78.

Chapter 4

Physical management of spasticity

Louise J Lockley and Katrina Buchanan

The individual with spasticity will hopefully benefit from the input of coordinated multidisciplinary care to effectively introduce and monitor a management plan for their spasticity with timely and appropriate interventions whenever necessary. The mainstay of a person's spasticity management will, however, occur at home and be carried out by themselves, with assistance perhaps from their family and carers. Encouragement, support and advice to maintain this work can enable the individual to successfully incorporate management techniques into their daily life, whatever their level of function. As outlined in Chapter 3, the two main components of this essential self-management are firstly the identification and moderation of any trigger or aggravating factors, and secondly the instigation of an effective and realistic physical programme, including attention to posture and positioning. Interestingly, despite the importance of carrying out physical strategies to help manage spasticity, many individuals do not have a regular physical programme in place. In a survey of over 20 000 people with multiple sclerosis (MS), 84% of participants reported spasticity; however, only just over half were using some form of physical therapy or stretching regime.[1]

The key to successful spasticity management is therefore through education of the individual to ensure that they understand and appreciate the importance of these factors. The use of written material to reinforce verbal information can be an effective method to facilitate this. Examples of both general spasticity information and advice to facilitate a home stretching programme are included in Appendices 3 and 4.

All members of the multidisciplinary team will be involved in providing education and support to the individual, and therefore it is essential that each health professional have a basic level of knowledge, including an appreciation of why positioning and movement are important as well as an understanding of available physical strategies that can be used to optimise an individual's overall spasticity management. The physiotherapist will of course be the key person to coordinate an appropriate physical management plan once a detailed assessment has been carried out (Chapter 2). Liaison between health and social care teams within both primary and secondary care will ensure that a consistent approach is maintained over time, with reinforcement to the individual and their family and carers about the aims and benefits of continuing a physical management programme. For instance, the need and time for a daily stretching programme can be successfully factored into the provision of a person's care package. Social service carers are taught how to perform stretches, which are then incorporated into their daily care routine when working with the person. Exploring provision of such models of practice with local care providers is extremely valuable.

It is also important for the team and the individual to appreciate that the degree, pattern and impact of spasticity on day-to-day function will vary over time.

As the spasticity changes, the appropriate physical intervention may also change, necessitating that any regime be flexible, with the opportunity to review and optimise the management plan at regular intervals.

SPASTICITY AND MOVEMENT

Muscle tone refers to the ongoing tension in a muscle, which is apparent as resistance experienced to passive movement and stretching. An increase in muscle tone or stiffness (hypertonia) can be due to an increase in the non-neural component due to altered viscoelastic properties of connective tissue and muscles crossing the joint or to changes within the joint itself, and in the neural component due predominantly to the stretch reflex. Hyperexcitability of stretch reflexes occurs due to alterations in the modulation of both ascending afferent signals (sensory information) and descending inhibitory pathways, either directly or via inhibitory spinal circuits (Chapter 1).

Stretch reflexes are an integral component to normal movement and function. Through their effect on limb stiffness, they are also important in the maintenance of posture. Modulation occurs according to task, with further changes throughout the different phases of movement. For example, during walking, stretch reflexes in the calf muscles may contribute to activation during push-off, be reduced during swing phase and then increase again during stance. This control of normal movement is vulnerable to any pathological changes in motor neuronal and spinal cord inhibitory interneuronal activity.

As well as hyperexcitable stretch reflexes causing an increase in muscle tone and reducing control of normal movement, the non-neural contribution to limb stiffness must not be forgotten. Connective tissue or joint changes can occur with or without contracture (irreversible changes in muscles, tendons and ligaments that result in loss of passive range at joints), and the resulting stiffness can vary in a velocity-dependent manner similar to spasticity, making it difficult to clinically distinguish between hypertonia of neural and non-neural origin.[2] This distinction is, however, clinically important, as the treatment of non-neural (or passive) stiffness is via physical adjuncts such as stretching and splinting and will not respond to pharmacological interventions. In addition to increased muscle tone by neural and non-neural mechanisms, people with spasticity will often display associated features, including spasms, clonus, associated reactions, positive support reactions and abnormal co-contraction (Chapter 1): all of these can further impact on normal patterns of movement and posture. Furthermore, it must be remembered that as well as these so-called positive features of the upper motor neurone (UMN) syndrome (Table 1.1), there are usually coexisting negative features such as weakness, reduced dexterity and fatigue. All of the components of the UMN syndrome, both positive and negative, may interact and contribute both to altered movement and to changes in the biomechanical properties of muscles, with the potential risk of contracture formation.

As different aspects of the UMN syndrome often occur in combination, it is essential to carry out a detailed assessment to identify the relative contribution each makes to an individual's reduction in function before initiating management plans (Chapter 2). However, on a practical note, as connective tissue and other non-neural changes almost invariably develop in the UMN syndrome, instigating an effective stretching and moving programme is a key component of any individual's management plan.

PHYSICAL MANAGEMENT STRATEGIES

The aims of a physical programme can be considered simply as maintaining or improving the current level of function while ensuring that future potential problems are avoided. The aim is not to reduce spasticity per se, as sometimes a person's function will be dependent on the presence of some increase in tone or possibly spasms – the focus must always be on function, reduction of pain or discomfort and on avoiding secondary complications such as contractures or adverse skin changes such as pressure sores.

The following key aims of a physical management programme can be considered an essential part of good general spasticity management:

- Minimise changes in the viscoelastic properties of connective tissue, muscles and joints, with the ultimate aim of maintaining range and preventing the development of contractures. This may be achieved by active and passive movement, standing, or stretching, or through the use of splints.
- Change patterns of spasticity or spasms to prevent them becoming self-perpetuating. For example, if

extensor tone and spasms are a dominant problem in the legs (stiff straight legs), then using a wedge or T-roll under the knees for night-time positioning may inhibit this pattern (by promoting a flexed position of the legs) and impact beneficially on the person's function and/or ease of care in the morning.

- Maintain or improve the person's level of function. A strengthening programme as well as considering cardiovascular fitness may be relevant.
- Recognise when and how spasticity or its associated features are useful functionally to a person, but prevent this use from reinforcing patterns of spasticity or contributing to increases in non-neural tone.

In addition to these general aims, there will be specific physical interventions that are indicated following changes in management. For example, in conjunction with botulinum toxin injections, an intensive physiotherapy and splinting programme may be instigated to maximise the benefit from the treatment. Likewise, following intrathecal therapies, there may be sudden dramatic changes in underlying spasticity or spasms, which will necessitate a full assessment, introduction of a new physical management plan and review of seating requirements.

In general, it is not just a single therapeutic intervention but a range of physical techniques that are incorporated into the management plan to achieve the best results. The range of therapeutic options used is outlined in Figure 4.1 and then discussed in turn in the following pages. Careful assessment and measurement will guide the decision-making process and allow for monitoring of the benefits gained.

STANDING

Standing has been used for many years as a physiotherapeutic intervention in people with neurological conditions and is acknowledged as forming an integral part of their rehabilitation and long-term management.[3] Its value was highlighted in the management of spasticity in the spinal injuries population as early as the 1970s[4] and since then has been the focus of several research studies in other conditions, with beneficial results.[5–10] The usefulness of assisted standing has been recognised in the Department of Health National Institute for Clinical Excellence (NICE) guidelines.[11]

Figure 4.1

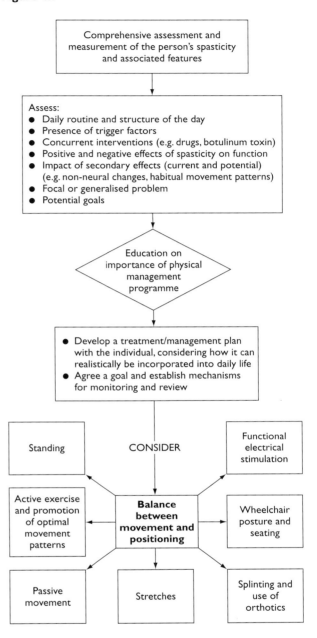

Process for selecting appropriate physical modalities for the individual with spasticity

Evidence base for standing

Research studies investigating the effects of standing have focused mainly on the use of the tilt table and have included individuals with varied neurological conditions, including spinal cord injury, acquired brain injury, cerebral palsy, stroke and MS. The results of these studies suggest beneficial effects of standing, with changes in passive range of movement, spasticity (as measured by the Ashworth scale), psychological well-being (by self-report) and neurophysiological measures; however, the sample sizes were small.[5–7,9,10,12] One further study considered the use of a motorised standing frame in six people with long-standing paraparesis. This study failed to show a benefit in scores of passive range of movement or spasticity, although interestingly individuals reported a benefit in general well-being and continued to stand regularly following completion of the study.[8]

Three self-report surveys have confirmed the subjective benefits of standing in larger sample sizes of individuals with spinal cord injury or MS.[13–15] Perceived benefits of standing included improved bladder and bowel function, a reduction in the incidence of urinary tract infections, reductions in spasticity and spasms, and fewer pressure sores. A significant proportion of participants also reported a positive psychological benefit, including improved self-esteem, self-image and morale. Reported side-effects were minor, with only a small proportion of people experiencing dizziness and/or fatigue.

The mechanisms responsible for the observed beneficial effects of standing in spasticity management are clearly complex, but are postulated to include the following:

- promotion of anti-gravity muscle activity in the trunk and lower limbs[3,16]
- maintenance or improvement in soft tissue and joint flexibility, thereby reducing the risk of contracture development[6]
- modulation of the neural component of spasticity through prolonged stretch and altered sensory input[5,7,10]
- reduction of lower-limb spasms[5]
- a positive psychological effect[8,14,15]

How long to stand for?

When looking for guidance from the literature regarding the optimum time and frequency for standing, it is clear that there is a lack of conclusive evidence. The duration of standing in reported studies varies from 30 minutes to a maximum of 1½ hours daily, often starting with shorter times and building up. From the results of the self-report surveys, it appears that individuals were standing on average for 40 minutes, three or four times a week.[13–15]

In practice, advice on standing regimes is individualised to the person and their lifestyle. Whenever possible, we encourage individuals who are predominantly wheelchair users or who spend the majority of the day in a sitting position to stand daily. This may

Figure 4.2

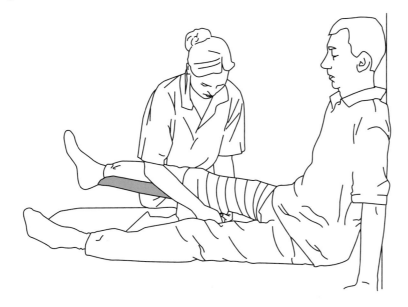

Application of a back slab in a long-sitting position

only be for a few minutes – but if achievable, half an hour would seem a reasonable target.

Ways to incorporate standing into the management plan

The optimal standing position is in an extended posture with neutral alignment of the trunk, pelvis and lower-limb joints. Careful assessment is needed to determine how this is best achieved and how it may be incorporated into an individual's daily routine. Optimising safety and posture in standing can be achieved through use of the environment or with specialised equipment.

Household equipment

People who are able to stand independently should be encouraged to do so at regular intervals throughout the day. In situations where the person has difficulty maintaining an optimal standing position (perhaps due to fatigue), resting their arms on a support such as a kitchen work surface, table or a walking aid can be helpful. For those in whom balance is compromised or who have proximal muscle weakness, for example around the trunk and pelvis, a surface behind such as a wall or worktop can also be beneficial.

Lower-limb splints

Using a custom-made hard splint such as a back slab[3] bandaged onto one or both of the lower limbs, or orthoses such as gaiters or knee-ankle-foot orthoses (KAFO), can be helpful if a person has muscle weakness leading to difficulty straightening their leg from the hip and/or knee. It can also be useful in situations where truncal and pelvic weakness impacts on the person's ability to extend the hips, often resulting in a posture of hyperextension or flexion at the knees. These splints are most easily applied with the person in a long-sitting position (Figure 4.2); care must be taken to check the skin before and after use. The disadvantage of these splints is that the person has to come up into a standing position in general, with the splinted leg or legs straight; therefore a manual handling risk assessment is essential. In people with good upper-body strength, this is usually less problematic; however, the use of a raised surface to stand from (e.g. a height-adjustable bed) may be helpful for all individuals and reduces risk.

Oswestry standing frame

This is a wooden frame with an integral table and straps that support the heels, knees and hips (Figure 4.3). Trunk support is also possible with the addition of a chest strap or with the use of a positioning wedge placed on the table. This type of frame can be used within a person's home and is particularly useful for people with lower-limb weakness where maintenance of an optimal standing position is difficult. In some parts of the UK, social service departments or community therapy teams may be able to lend standing frames to individuals. Other facilities where this equipment may be available include day centres and MS centres.

Motorised or hydraulically assisted standing systems

A mechanical or electrically powered standing frame can be useful if a person is unable to stand up from

Figure 4.3

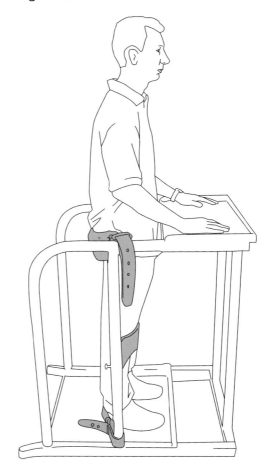

Standing in an Oswestry standing frame

sitting independently (Figure 4.4). This device moves the person into a standing position, and once they are upright supports the hips, knees and ankles. Additional truncal support is also usually possible. In some models, a person with good upper-body strength can operate the equipment themselves; however, in most situations, some assistance is generally required with set-up.

Standing wheelchair

Standing wheelchairs are becoming more widely available and often provide the easiest means for a person who is wheelchair-dependent to stand regularly during the day. Some are electrically powered, while others have a manual hydraulic system, with the lifting device fitted as an integral part of the chair. The benefits of these standing systems are that a person can incorporate standing into everyday tasks, such as getting items out of cupboards or cleaning their teeth, and they can in general operate them without the need for assistance. The drawbacks are that in some models, the chair is mechanically unable to reach a fully upright standing position, preventing

Figure 4.4

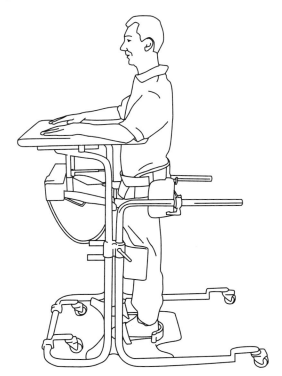

Standing in a motorised frame (Quest 88 pictured)

the person's hips extending to the neutral position; also, the additional weight of the mechanism can make the chair heavier to propel.

It is always beneficial for the individual to trial standing in one of these systems before committing to a specific product; this can usually be arranged directly with the suppliers.

Tilt table

A tilt table is generally only used when none of the above options are possible and the person needs maximum support throughout the body to stand (Figure 4.5). It is a particularly useful adjunct in the acute stages of a neurological condition or if a person has not stood for a long time. In both situations, postural hypotension may be a concern, and the tilt table allows for a rapid return to a supine position should this occur. Standing with a tilt table requires no active participation from the individual, allowing it to be used even in the presence of significant generalised muscle weakness. It can sometimes be impossible to achieve full extension at the hips; however, if a person is confined to bed or spending prolonged periods of time in a flexed position then the use of the tilt table gives significantly more extension throughout the body and allows some weight to be put through the feet.

Implementing a standing programme

Where possible, standing is recommended as part of the 24-hour management programme for people with spasticity. Careful assessment and trial of equipment can ensure that the person is able to stand with optimal alignment for a sustained period of time, both comfortably and safely and in a way that allows them to utilise their muscle activity to the maximum. The main barrier to standing is frequently access to equipment, which can be costly and will require regular maintenance. Exploring novel funding mechanisms through local or national charitable organisations, or workplaces, or factoring the cost into health packages can be useful.

It is vitally important to educate individuals and, if appropriate, their families or carers about the optimal posture for standing and how this is most easily achieved. Techniques to minimise spasms when rising from sitting to standing, such as moving slowly and allowing time for the person to accommodate to the stretch before standing fully upright, are useful.

Figure 4.5

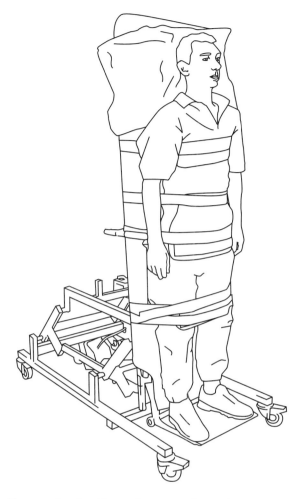

The use of a tilt table to allow a standing position

Routinely checking for any skin changes before and after standing is also recommended to monitor potentially vulnerable areas such as behind the knees and under the feet.

The effects of standing, both positive and negative, should be monitored over time by the person with spasticity as well as the relevant health professionals or team; modifications can then be made to the programme as the need arises.

ACTIVE EXERCISE AND PROMOTION OF OPTIMAL MOVEMENT PATTERNS

Where possible, active exercise to increase strength, re-educate movement patterns and improve cardiovascular fitness should be encouraged, as the effects are greater than those seen with passive exercise alone.

Historically, physiotherapy treatments in individuals with the UMN syndromes were primarily aimed at reducing spasticity, with the hope that this would increase function. Little attention was given to the role of muscle weakness, and in fact strength training was often avoided due to the fear of exacerbating spasticity. However, more recently, there has been an increased understanding of the interactions of the different aspects of the UMN syndrome, with awareness that muscles with spasticity and their antagonists may all be weak, but there is invariably relative overactivity of one versus the other.[17] This imbalance between agonist and antagonist activity often impairs functional movement and in turn may lead to muscle atrophy, soft tissue changes and ultimately joint deformity.

All skeletal muscles have adaptive potential and are therefore capable of modifying their structure in response to environmental changes, which may be beneficial or detrimental to function.[18] This capacity means that with appropriate and specific training, muscle has the ability to modify its structure and function enabling such imbalances between agonist and antagonist pairs to be minimised.[18] This process can sometimes be further facilitated by using pharmacological means (botulinum toxin) to weaken an overactive muscle, allowing strength training of its antagonist, with the aim of improving function (Chapter 6).

Changing/re-educating patterns of movement

It is clear that altered patterns of activity can affect muscle structure and function. Individuals with spasticity and spasms are often forced into stereotypical movement patterns, which are then reinforced by the subsequent soft tissue change, leaving certain muscle groups at a biomechanical disadvantage. Where possible, it is beneficial to encourage active movement in combination with appropriate stretching to establish more efficient movement and maintenance of muscle balance. It is important not to neglect the trunk and pelvis within this process, as proximal control is crucial as a basis for limb function, with alignment and strength of the trunk and pelvis having a significant impact on both spasms and spasticity.

Using spasticity or spasms to aid function

In some situations, spasticity and spasms can be extremely helpful for function; however, continued use of stereotypical patterns can lead to permanent biomechanical changes in the soft tissues. It is important to establish whether such strategies are essential to a particular function or are the only means by which someone with significant weakness can move. For example, it is not uncommon for people to use an extensor spasm in their legs to assist in standing from sitting or to rely on a straight leg to stand on while stepping. Despite the usefulness of such strategies, it is very important that the individual have an understanding of the possible consequences of utilising their spasticity or spasms in this way, enabling them to prevent further complications.

Evidence base for strengthening programmes

The change in attitude with respect to the value of strengthening muscles in individuals with significant spasticity has been aided by its evaluation in several research studies. A systematic review of the effectiveness of strength-training programmes for people with cerebral palsy carried out by Dodd et al[19] analysed the results of 11 studies and reported no evidence of negative effects such as reduced range of motion or increasing spasticity. Positive effects were seen, with increased strength and improvements in motor function.

These beneficial effects were confirmed in a further study of 10 people with cerebral palsy who underwent 10 weeks of strength training twice a week lasting 1 hour in duration, compared with controls who were not exercising. The results demonstrated significant improvements in the exercise group in muscle strength, gross motor function, walking velocity and timed up-and-go, with no evidence of increased spasticity.[20]

Further studies of strength training have been carried out in the stroke population; these have been reviewed, with positive effects being demonstrated in both lower-limb strength and walking speed.[21] Similarly, in a small study in MS, a strengthening programme was shown to have beneficial effects on both fatigue and walking ability.[22]

Strength training in practice

Clearly, a strengthening programme requires commitment from the person and therefore needs to be realistic for the individual to fit into their daily life. Including training that is task-specific such as sit-to-stand or step-ups is beneficial and also may be more easily incorporated into the daily routine.

Factors to bear in mind with strength training include consideration of muscle length, velocity of movement, the use of task-based training (e.g. sit-to-stand), training load, number of repetitions and intensity (times per week). Traditional training rates are a load of 60–80% of one repetition maximum (the maximum load that can be lifted once), three sets of 10 repetitions carried out three or four times a week; however, these parameters are based on the sports literature and it is not clear whether they are optimal for all people with neurological conditions.

When devising programmes, it is important to consider all affected muscle groups, including those in which spasticity is present, to prevent any further imbalances that may predispose the individual to develop abnormal movement patterns. Careful positioning is also essential to ensure the safety, comfort and specificity of training without triggering spasticity or spasms.

Cardiovascular fitness

Maintaining good general health is of course important for everyone; however, it can be a neglected area, particularly in people who have limited mobility. There is evidence within the MS population that regular aerobic exercise reduces fatigue and increases strength, walking speed, and physical and psychological well-being.[23,24] Likewise, the Cochrane review promotes the benefits of exercise therapy in MS, with no evidence of deleterious effects; it states that exercise therapy should be advocated in all patients when they are not experiencing an exacerbation.[25]

A review of the value of cardiovascular exercise in people with stroke, suggests that this may positively influence walking speed and distance.[21]

PASSIVE MOVEMENTS

Passive movement utilises external assistance from a second person or a mechanical aid to move the limb in situations where active movement is not possible or significantly increases spasticity or spasms. As part of a passive movement programme, it is recommended that all affected body parts be moved through their available range of motion on a daily basis.

Evidence for the use of passive movements is limited; however, they continue to be recommended by clinicians on the basis of the physiological assumption that movement is beneficial to change patterns of spasticity, combat secondary non-neural changes and facilitate optimal positioning. Instigating a passive movement programme before tasks such as washing and dressing can facilitate care and increase comfort.

Evidence base

In a small study of seven brain-injured hemiparetic people, Schmit et al[26] demonstrated a reduction in elbow flexor stretch reflexes after repeated large-amplitude joint movements, indicating a significant short-term beneficial reduction in spastic hypertonia following passive movement.

Similarly, passive movement at the knee in stroke patients has been shown to reduce electromyography (EMG) activity and torque measures in both the flexors and extensors of the knee: this was thought to be due to a combination of reflex and non-neural (viscoelastic) factors.[27] Interestingly, in both studies, the largest changes were seen after the first movement: it remains unclear whether the effects are sustainable over time.

Passive cycling is an attractive means of passive movement as it does not require a second person apart from perhaps in set-up. Two studies have investigated its effect on spasticity: one in people with MS and the other in spinal cord injury. Unfortunately, neither study showed any definite change in spasticity (assessed by neurophysiological measures and torque using a dynamometer); however, participants reported a subjective beneficial effect on their spasticity.[28,29]

Incorporating passive movements into the 24-hour management plan

Consideration of how passive movements can be incorporated in the daily routine is essential to ensure their continued use on a day-to-day basis. It may be possible to teach a relative or carer to include them in the morning care regime or to carry out a few movements prior to repositioning, for example when placing a T-roll between the legs or when the person with spasticity is being moved from bed to chair. Care should be taken with the position of both the person and their assistant to allow for comfort, ease of movement and safety. Timing anti-spasticity medication so that it is taken 20–30 minutes before the movements are carried out will give the maximum benefit for both parties involved.

Movements should be performed at a slow speed to avoid causing trauma to the muscles and to minimise triggering of the stretch reflex. Spasms may occur secondary to the sensory or stretch stimuli: if this is problematic, the movement should be halted and continued once the spasm passes. If the skin is very sensitive to touch then a gradual programme of handling may help to desensitise the skin; alternatively, handling the limb on top of clothes may help. It is often helpful to avoid holding the ball of the foot, as this sensory stimulation can be a common trigger for spasms.

Generally, passive movements are carried out with the person lying down; however, the upper limbs and back can also be moved with the person in a sitting or supported standing position. Starting positions can influence the level of tone or occurrence of spasms: for example, if the person experiences extensor spasms in their legs when lying flat, the use of a positioning aid such as a T-roll, pillows or bed mechanism to bend the knees prior to starting the movements can reduce the number of spasms. Movements should always be carried out in optimal alignments of the muscles and joints to avoid trauma, while avoiding overstretching (this can damage muscles and skin, particularly in the vulnerable areas behind the knees or in elbow creases) and stereotypical spasticity patterning (e.g. flexing the hip in midline rather than in adduction and internal rotation).

It is important that once the movements are completed the benefits are not lost by ensuring that the person is positioned appropriately afterwards, avoiding typical positions adopted as a result of their spasticity or spasms.

In most healthcare settings, health professionals may not be able to carry out passive movements regularly due to time and funding constraints. It may, however, be possible to incorporate a passive movement programme into a person's care package. In most cases, passive movements are carried out on an ongoing basis by families, carers or friends: it is extremely important that these people have access to education about how to implement an appropriate programme. Teaching passive movements correctly is vitally important to ensure that no damage is done to the person or their carer and that the movements are effective. The individual and their families or carers should also have knowledge of how to access health professionals should any problems arise or if the spasticity changes.

Adjuncts to passive movement

Equipment that can be used to assist with passive movements includes continuous passive movement machines (CPM) to flex and extend a limb, or passive cycles, which the person can use from a sitting position. Hoisting can also provide a means of flexing the lower limbs and trunk: therefore, in circumstances where opportunities for passive movement are limited, regular position changes using the hoist may be beneficial. Due to the risk of skin trauma and discomfort, it is not advisable for the person to be left in the hoist for a prolonged period of time.

STRETCHES

It is well known that immobilisation of a muscle in a shortened position causes muscle atrophy, fibre shortening and reduced muscle compliance, with an increase in the ratio of collagen to muscle fibre tissue.[17] These histological changes are detectable within as little as 2 days after the onset of immobilisation. The muscle fibre shortening and reduced compliance can in turn increase spindle sensitivity in response to stretch, thus also exacerbating neural changes (spasticity), which can of course predispose the individual to further non-neural changes.[30]

Muscles are, however, adaptive, and maintained stretch is a signal for the production of additional actin and myosin filaments as well as new sarcomeres.[17,31] Stretching is therefore a therapeutic means by which to maintain or increase muscle length.

Evidence base

Although several studies have looked at the effects of stretching on range of movement, there is little agreement on how long stretches should be held for or how frequently they should be performed.

In animal studies, stretches for only 30 minutes have been advocated to be sufficient to prevent loss of muscle sarcomeres.[32] Conversely, in human studies, it has been suggested that time periods of a minimum of 6 hours are necessary to prevent contracture formation.[33] A study has demonstrated that 30 minutes of calf muscle stretching daily was sufficient to maintain but not increase range at the ankle; however, the results may have been influenced by the fact that some of the participants were positioned with their ankles at plantargrade while in the wheelchair, providing further

sustained stretching.[34] A further small study found no benefit from 30 minutes of stretching twice daily in preventing contractures in the upper limb post stroke.[35]

The effect of stretching on spasticity has attracted little attention in the literature. So called 'anti-spastic positioning' has been utilised in children with cerebral palsy as part of an exercise plan to prevent contractures or deformities. The aim is to keep muscles in a lengthened position for as long as tolerable, with the hope of desensitisation of stretch receptors by the prolonged and slow stretching. In a study of 20 children with spastic diplegia positioned for 20 minutes (upright sitting with hip abduction and external rotation, knee extension and ankle dorsiflexion), reductions in spasticity as measured by EMG, the modified Ashworth scale and goniometry were seen.[36] However, it remains unclear from the literature how long this positioning should be held and for how long the beneficial effects last.

Incorporating stretching into the 24-hour management plan

When formulating a stretching programme, it is important to consider the person's daily routine and posture throughout the day. Stretches can be carried out both actively and passively (with assistance from another person incorporated into a passive range of movement routine or using adjuncts such as functional electrical stimulation (FES)). Periods of prolonged stretch can be achieved by positioning, including standing, sitting and lying and also via the use of splints or orthotics. It must, however, be remembered that stretching one muscle puts the opposing muscle group in a position of relative shortening. It is therefore important that stretching regimes be balanced and aim for optimal alignment for function.

There is no clear direction from the literature about how long a muscle needs to be stretched to prevent or reverse contracture, but longer periods of time appear to be more effective. In addition, stretching can be particularly beneficial prior to exercise and may actually improve the activation of muscles. This is demonstrated by a study in children with cerebral palsy, who following stretching showed an improved range of active hip abduction.[37]

Provision of an information sheet depicting common stretches can be very useful in educating individuals about why certain stretches are useful. An example of an advice sheet regarding stretching is included in Appendix 4.

This leaflet can be easily individualised by the therapist ticking the relevant exercises and indicating both the frequency and duration for which each stretch should be performed.

POSITIONING

Through careful positioning, muscles can be held in a lengthened state enabling a sustained stretch; this can be used as a means to maintain or increase range of movement.

The use of optimal positioning is an important feature in the management of spasticity in all individuals – from those with mild tightening of a calf when waking in the morning to those with severe generalised spasticity.

The general benefits of positioning are to:

- allow lengthening of vulnerable soft tissues in a variety of positions throughout the day and night
- change patterns of spasticity and reduce spasms by positioning in postures opposite to the pattern of the spasticity or spasms (e.g. if extensor spasms are problematic then position in flexion)
- correct asymmetry, particularly of the spine and pelvis, which can be influenced by limb position – for example, wind sweeping of the legs will cause rotation of the pelvis
- support the body in a comfortable position to allow relaxation and acceptance of the base of support

The key to successful positioning regimes is regular changing of positions throughout the day. Maintaining one position all the time not only is uncomfortable and potentially dangerous (putting the person at risk of reduced skin integrity) but also puts those muscles that are not in a lengthened position at risk of shortening and developing contractures.

Optimising positioning is important in all postures from lying to standing, and when assessing the impact of spasticity on a person's life, it is vital to look at the effect of all positions on their spasticity. The presence of trigger or aggravating factors (e.g. pressure sores, pain or discomfort) will all influence the

options for positioning. If a posture is comfortable then it will maximise muscle relaxation, and this will facilitate the stretch and enable a person to stay in the position for a longer period of time.

Passive exercise can be helpful before positioning to reduce stiffness: for example, if extensor tone is problematic, bending the hips and knees up towards the chest a few times can help when positioning the legs into flexion using a positioning aid such as a T-roll.

For positioning to be effective, the affected muscle groups should be placed in more of a lengthened position than they naturally fall into. For example, if a person has increased bilateral hip adductor tone and their knees are constantly held together then the following approaches can be adopted to change this position:

- The person can monitor the position of their knees when sitting, trying to keep them apart to prevent adduction becoming a habitual resting pattern.
- Investigate the impact of trunk and pelvis position on the legs. If the person is sitting in a flexed posture with a posteriorly tilted pelvis, this can cause the legs to rest in an internally rotated and adducted position. Having a firmer seat base, a contoured cushion or an extra trunk support may facilitate a more anteriorly tilted position of the pelvis, extension of the trunk, and better lower-limb alignment.
- Instigate a daily hip adductor stretch programme.
- If a person is unable to monitor and/or change the position of their legs then aids such as a pummel, rolled-up towel or cushion placed between the knees to maintain some length of the hip adductors can be helpful. A T-roll can be very effective in bed for the same reasons.

Equipment to aid positioning

- T-rolls and wedges can be used to maintain a flexed position at the knees and hips and bring the lumbar spine into more flexion, which in turn can reduce extensor spasticity and spasms (Figures 4.6 and 4.7). In addition, these positioning aids promote more equal loading of the tissues and improve alignment of the body segments.[16] An added benefit of T-rolls compared with wedges is to provide a stretch to the hip adductors, which can impact on hip adductor tone; this effect is

Figure 4.6

(a)

(b)

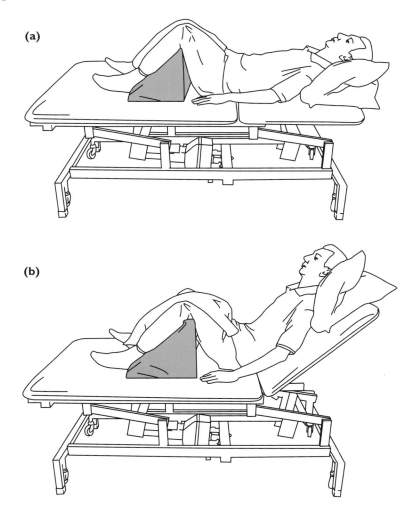

The use of a wedge in lying (a) and sitting (b)

Figure 4.7

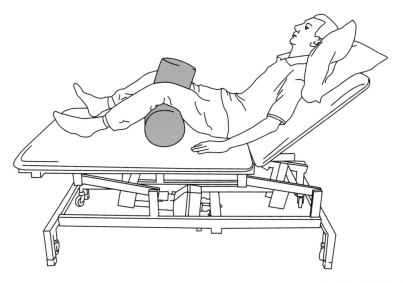

The use of a T-roll in sitting

preserved when using the T-roll in side-lying (Figure 4.8). Care is needed with any positioning aid when spasms are present, as there is the potential for skin trauma or pressure areas to develop.

- Everyday items such as pillows and towels can be used if more expensive equipment is unavailable or unhelpful.
- Electrically powered profiling beds can be used to help position a person in flexion or long-sitting if extensor tone and spasms are problematic.
- Trays and tables can be helpful to position the upper limb.
- Physiotherapists may sometimes use large gym balls to assist in breaking whole-body extensor tone. The person with spasticity is placed over the ball so that flexion is introduced throughout the body. This can be very helpful, but requires careful handling skills, with generally more than one therapist and sometimes a hoist.
- Specialised sleeping systems can be helpful when other equipment to promote positioning during sleep is no longer effective or supportive in a position that allows relaxation.

Figure 4.8

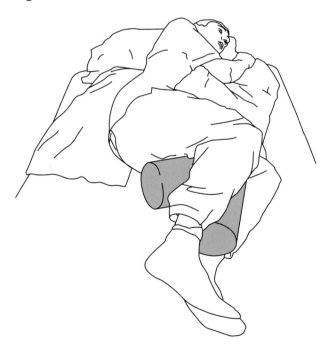

The use of a T-roll in side-lying

WHEELCHAIR AND SEATING FOR PEOPLE WITH SPASTICITY

For individuals who depend on a wheelchair for their mobility or who may be spending the majority of their waking hours in their chair, posture and seating are of paramount importance.

A thorough assessment of an individual's spasticity is necessary before advising on the most appropriate seating. This will help differentiate tone that is problematic for posture and function from that which may be useful and may be used to enhance motor patterns for functional purposes. Hypertonia itself may allow the maintenance of a sitting posture, particularly in those individuals with significant truncal weakness; however, it may also lead to problems of postural instability, reduced upper-limb function and joint contractures.[38] Optimal positioning of a person via the use of an appropriate seating system can assist in reducing these problems and will help maximise function.[39,40]

Goals of seating in patients with spasticity

- Facilitate function – for example improved use of head and upper limbs
- Reduce the risk of biomechanical changes in muscles, tendons and joints that can impact on health and hygiene
- Accommodate to contractures or bony deformities that may already be established
- Increase comfort
- Minimise effects of fatigue on posture
- Reduce work of breathing and improve quality of speech

Careful assessment of the individual is of utmost importance: the best way to determine a person's optimum position is with a hands-on evaluation in both supine and sitting positions.[39] This allows an assessment of the person's physical abilities and limitations, the opportunity to mimic postures, and the identification of areas where support may be needed. It is important to consider any triggers for spasticity or spasms, including positions that may influence these. Generally, when the person is in a comfortable and well-supported position, tone and spasms will be minimised.

Improving proximal stability can often make a dramatic difference to an individual's level of function, as it provides a fixed origin from which muscles can work more effectively. For example, a well-aligned pelvis provides a stable base for the spine so that the neck and head are free to move more precisely. The fundamental stabilising feature of a seating system is a firm seat base and back rest, and subtle changes to this may impact on a person's posture and spasticity. This can be illustrated by altering the seat base to promote a slight anterior tilt of the pelvis: this assists in reducing extensor tone by encouraging hip flexion, abduction and external rotation as well as extension of the trunk. Similarly, in people with weak trunks and neck extensors, reclining the back rest slightly allows gravity to hold the upper trunk and head against the posterior supporting surfaces. This reduces the workload of the muscles and can reduce spasticity and spasms in the trunk and limbs. However, it is important to consider that changes in one aspect of a seating system may influence others: by reclining the back rest, flexion at the hips may be reduced, which can cause problems with extensor tone. Often, if possible, a tilt-in-space chair is the best option, as it tips the entire seating system back, not just the backrest, thus avoiding extension at the hip joints. Tilt-in-space options have also been found to improve respiration and reduce kyphosis for people with various neurological conditions; in addition, reduction in effort or work of speaking and breathing for people with MS has been reported.[41]

Additional supports such as head rests and tables can help reduce the risk of fatigue impacting on postural alignment by supporting the weight of the head and arms. Frequent rests from the upright sitting position using the tilt-in-space mechanism can also help with managing fatigue and redistributing pressure. Some people will benefit greatly from the use of static seating systems (e.g. Kirton chairs) that have a tilt-in-space mechanism and adjustments to allow leg position to be changed.

Over the course of time, levels of function and spasticity may change: this is particularly evident after therapeutic interventions such as alterations in drug management, including the use of intrathecal baclofen or phenol. It is therefore extremely important that seating needs be reviewed regularly and promptly, especially after any treatment interventions. Ideally, before intrathecal therapies that are expected to have a major impact on seating requirements are carried out, liaison should be established between seating clinics and the multidisciplinary team.

SPLINTING AND THE USE OF ORTHOSES

An orthosis or splint is an external device designed to apply, distribute or remove forces to or from the body in a controlled manner to perform one or both of the basic functions of:[42]

- control of body motion
- alteration or prevention of alteration in the shape of the body tissues

It is common practice for clinicians to refer to orthoses as those external devices usually custom-made by an orthotist. The term 'splint' is usually reserved for devices made from low-temperature plastics or fabric by therapists. Non-removable splinting devices made of plaster or casting tape are referred to as 'casts'. However, within the literature and clinical practice, the terms 'splint', 'cast' and 'orthosis' are often used interchangeably.

Splints or orthotics are rarely used in isolation; however, they can be useful adjuncts to therapy in the following ways:

- to provide a means of controlling the range of movement around a joint and thereby facilitate function
- to apply a prolonged stretch to a muscle to prevent or correct soft tissue changes
- to compensate for deformity (e.g. a heel raise to compensate for leg length discrepancy)
- as a means of modulating the neural component of spasticity through prolonged stretch and altered sensory input
- to increase comfort

Evidence base

Splints and casts

The use of casts in the management of hypertonia was first described in the 1960s in children with cerebral palsy, and in more recent years, it has been advocated in adults with a variety of neurological conditions but in particular brain injury.

In 1998, the Association of Chartered Physiotherapists Interested in Neurology (ACPIN) reviewed the splinting evidence base and wrote clinical practice guidelines for splinting adults with neurological dysfunction.[43] These guidelines highlighted the lack of evidence in relation to splinting regimes, including timing of intervention, length of application and the effect of stretch on muscle length. They did, however, provide guidance on the use of splints in clinical practice, and this has been expanded on in certain texts.[3]

Since the production of these guidelines, a further systematic review of the literature in relation to the effects of casting on passive range of motion, spasticity and function in adults post head injury has been completed. This review analysed 13 studies, all conducted within inpatient hospital settings.[44] Casting was recognised as not being the sole intervention, and in general was carried out in combination with rehabilitation including anti-spasticity medication. Out of these 12 studies, only five measured spasticity as an outcome, the remaining studies looked at passive range of motion and functional measures. All of the studies reported improvement to some extent in the level of spasticity post casting, although no validated outcome measures were used. Changes in passive range of motion were seen, with maintenance of or an increase in passive range being demonstrated.[44] Due to the variation in splinting regimes, particularly in terms of duration of application, there is no clear guidance from the literature with regard to the optimal time to splint for, the number of different casts needed or whether to use removable or non-removable splints.

A recent study has investigated the effects of casting on ankle range of movement, with and without the additional use of botulinum toxin, in people with acute severe brain injury.[45] Below knee removable (combination soft/scotch cast) splints were custom-made within the first 2 weeks of injury. The results demonstrated that casting was more effective than regular physiotherapy in maintaining range of motion, but there was no additional benefit when combined with botulinum toxin. However, in the casting group, four out of the 12 people required rescue botulinum toxin treatment due to loss of range of movement, confounding interpretation of the results. The study highlights that the use of splinting in clinical practice requires skilled staff and ongoing monitoring, suggesting that in situations where this is not available, botulinum toxin may be the treatment of choice.[45] Further studies will be needed to determine the effect of combination treatment.

There have been relatively few studies investigating the use of hand splinting.[46] One randomised study considered overnight splinting of the hand in the functional position as a means of preventing contracture, reducing pain and improving function in 28 people with stroke.[47] This study concluded that there was insufficient evidence to either support or refute the effectiveness of hand splinting in people already participating in motor training combined with upper-limb stretches.[46]

Lycra has become a material of interest, particularly in the paediatric population, and more recently has been investigated in adults with hemiplegia. In a study of 16 adults with hemiplegic stroke, individually tailored Lycra wrist and hand splints were worn for 3 hours to encourage extension of the wrist and fingers, and supination of the forearm.[48] Results demonstrated improved wrist posture, reduced spasticity (measured by the Tardieu scale) in the wrist and fingers, improved passive range of motion at the shoulder, and reduced swelling in the hand; however, flexion of the fingers was restricted while the splint was in use.

Orthotics

There is a paucity of evidence for the use of orthotics in the management of spasticity. The majority of orthotic studies carried out make reference to spasticity, but in general look at functional measures such as gait or passive range of motion as their outcome. One study investigated the effect of an inhibitor bar attached to an ankle–foot orthosis (AFO) in stroke patients as a means of modulating tone. The modified Ashworth scale was used in addition to gait measures, and results showed no significant differences in spasticity; however, improved speed, stride length and cadence of gait were seen.[49] A Cochrane review[50] is currently underway to determine the effectiveness of the use of orthotic devices in the upper and lower limbs following stroke and non-progressive causes of spasticity. This is focusing on managing problems arising from spasticity, improving function and preventing complications.

The National Clinical Guidelines for Stroke[51] advocate that customised AFOs should be considered for people with foot drop to optimise their walking ability. The guidelines also propose the use of serial casting to prevent or reverse contractures and to reduce spasticity. Similarly, the NICE MS guidelines[11] suggest that in people with spasticity and spasms, the use of splints and serial casting should be considered.

Clinical uses

The use of splints in people with hypertonia requires careful assessment and monitoring to ensure suitability and effectiveness. Obtaining informed consent prior to the use of any splint or orthosis is essential; specific information needs to be provided with regard to risks and anticipated benefits. If the splint is uncomfortable, tone may be exacerbated and the person will be at risk of impaired skin integrity. If the splint is of suboptimal fit, there is the additional risk of secondary musculoskeletal deformity.

Essential considerations to take into account before using or making a splint are detailed in Table 4.1. There are no absolute contraindications to splinting; however, in the presence of any of the precautions listed in Table 4.1, it is good practice to document concerns with a written plan of how best to manage these. For example, if the person has reduced sensation then a programme of regular checking of the skin combined with a graded wearing regime, starting with short periods of use and building up over time, needs to be put in place.

Splints used in clinical practice take on many forms, and can either be static or dynamic, prefabricated or customised for the individual. A wide variety of materials are used, including polyurethane-impregnated bandages (soft/scotch cast), thermo-plastic materials, neoprene, Lycra and woven or soft materials. Choice of material will depend on the weight of the splint, setting time, cost, durability, ease of application and removal, but can also be a matter of personal preference and experience of use.

The most frequently used splints or orthoses include:

- wrist/hand splints
- elbow splints
- AFOs, insoles and ankle supports
- knee splints – gaiters/callipers
- spinal braces, hip braces and neck collars

Wrist and hand splints

Wrist and hand splints can be made from a variety of materials, including thermoplastic material, soft/scotch cast, neoprene, Lycra or woven/sheepskin materials.

Indications for use include:

- maintenance of range of movement: for example, a resting splint can be used to preserve optimal soft tissue length and joint alignment (Figure 4.9)
- facilitating function: for example, a wrist splint may promote a better grip while feeding by

Table 4.1 Indications and precautions for the use of splints or orthoses

Indications	Precautions
• Maintain joint range, soft tissue length and alignment	• Sensory impairment
• Increase soft tissue length and passive range of movement	• Unstable intracranial pressure
• Facilitate function (e.g. ankle-foot orthosis)	• Poor skin condition
• Facilitate hygiene (e.g. by enabling access to palm)	• Vascular disorder
• Increase comfort (e.g. sheepskin palm protector, Figure 4.11)	• Fracture or severe soft tissue injury
	• Behavioural/cognitive disorders
	• Uncontrolled epilepsy
	• Heterotrophic ossification
	• Oedema
	• Acute inflammation
	• Access to limb required for medical purposes
	• Medically unstable
	• Frequent spasms

supporting the wrist in an optimal position (Figure 4.10) or allow for targeted practice of finger extension

- maintaining hygiene: for example, a sheepskin palm protector can be used (Figure 4.11)

Elbow splints

Elbow splints are generally used in situations where there is the potential to lose range of movement or where range of movement has already been lost. This can be due to increased tone in the biceps muscle keeping the arm in a flexed position or to the unopposed action of the biceps in a cervical cord injury. These types of splints are frequently made from a combination of soft/scotch cast or thermoplastic material. In some situations, foam wrapped circum-

ferentially around the limb and secured with bandages can be useful – in particular when skin integrity, frequent spasms or dysautonomia may be problematic (Figure 4.12).[52]

Foot and ankle splints

Foot and ankle splints can be used as a means of reducing the range of movement around the ankle joint to facilitate function. An AFO or soft/scotch cast below-knee splint can maintain a dropped foot in a plantargrade or if possible a slightly dorsiflexed position to improve the efficiency of walking (Figure 4.13). Other foot and ankle splints can be used as a means of maintaining or increasing the range of movement at the ankle. Both serial casting (non-removable) and combination (removable) splints have

Figure 4.9

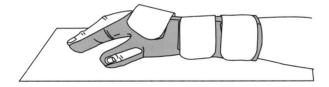

A resting hand splint made from soft/scotch cast materials, maintaining the interphalangeal joints of the fingers in extension, with flexion at the metacarpophalangeal joints and the thumb in a position of relative opposition

Figure 4.10

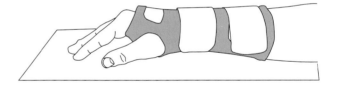

Wrist splint made from soft/scotch cast materials

Figure 4.11

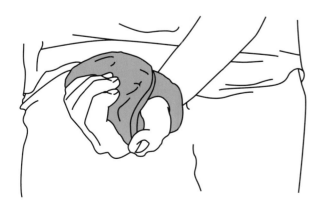

Sheepskin palm protector

Figure 4.12

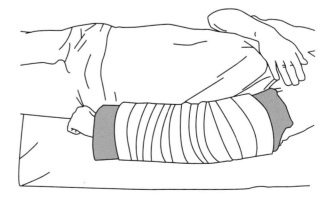

Foam elbow splint

Figure 4.13

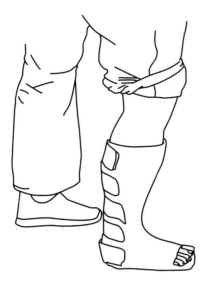

Below-knee splint made from soft/scotch cast to facilitate walking

been used as a means to achieve this with beneficial results; it is not clear from the literature which may be the preferred method. The use of non-removable casts ensures maintenance of the stretch position for a prolonged period of time, but does not allow for checking of the skin and can necessitate removal if oedema becomes an issue. Removable splints allow for regular checking of the skin and for removal of the splints for therapy or washing; however, the splints can sometimes be difficult to reapply in the optimal position if marked levels of spasticity are present. Removable splints also allow for tolerance to be built up gradually.

When making a splint with the aim of increasing range, the limb should not be splinted in the maximal-stretch position but slightly off this to minimise discomfort and thereby improve tolerance.

Knee splints

Knee splints can be used within function to facilitate a better standing position (e.g. backslabs: Figure 4.2, see the section on standing) or as a means of controlling the position of the knee while walking.

In situations where loss of range of motion at the knee is present, most frequently due to shortening in the hamstring muscles, combination soft/scotch cast

long leg casts can provide the most effective means of applying a prolonged stretch. Where there is minimal or no loss of range or when there are concerns regarding skin integrity or frequent spasms, foam splints can be more suitable (Figure 4.14).

Spinal braces

In general, these types of orthoses are made for the individual by an orthotist from polypropylene materials. They are often used to provide support to the spine and prevent secondary bony deformity in situations where there is muscle weakness. In individuals where spasticity is the overriding problem, spinal braces may not be suitable due to the significant muscular forces that can be present, which in turn may lead to problems with pressure areas. Spinal braces can also be difficult to fit, uncomfortable and impact on breathing. Use of customised seating with individualised truncal and pelvic support can be a more beneficial and comfortable option in these situations.

Splinting following the use of botulinum toxin

Splinting can be a useful adjunct following botulinum toxin to facilitate stretch and activity in the opposing muscle group. For example, following botulinum toxin injections into the wrist and finger flexors, a wrist splint may allow targeted practice of finger extension with the wrist in a neutral or slightly extended position. A potential goal for this intervention would be to enable the person to hold and release a cup, or alternatively to be able to stabilise their plate with the fingers in extension. Ideally, splints should be made 7–10 days post botulinum toxin to ensure that the maximum benefit of the toxin is gained.

Figure 4.14

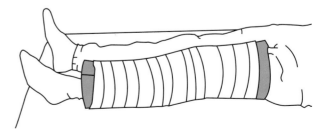

Lower-limb (knee) foam splint

Use of splinting and orthotics within a spasticity management programme

The use of splints in the management of people with neurological dysfunction can be a beneficial adjunct to other interventions; however, it should not be considered as a treatment in its own right. Careful assessment combined with goal setting and review of outcome is needed to ensure suitability of use. Where frequent spasms and significant levels of spasticity are present, splinting should be used with caution, and alternative types of splint that are less rigid (e.g. foam or sheepskin) should be explored. Combining splinting with oral medication, botulinum toxin or even intrathecal therapies may be indicated.

HYDROTHERAPY

Although access to a hydrotherapy pool may not be possible for many people, for those for whom it is it can be a beneficial intervention. People with spasticity, who find movement difficult, may find that the water enables them to move more freely. One study found that 20 minutes of hydrotherapy three times a week assisted in decreasing spasticity and spasm (measured by the Ashworth score) in spinal cord injury patients.[53] Immersion in warm water can provide body relaxation and postural support, allowing movement that may not be possible on land. However, not only can it be difficult to access a pool, it can also be difficult to find a pool that is at the right temperature. Both too cold or too warm water can exacerbate symptoms such as weakness and fatigue.

FUNCTIONAL ELECTRICAL STIMULATION

Functional electrical stimulation (FES) may be used to improve specific functions such as walking, to help strengthen weak muscles, as part of a stretching programme to maintain range of movement and potentially to reduce spasticity. FES was first used to improve the gait of patients with foot drop secondary to UMN lesions in the late 1950s and early 1960s.[54] However, mainly due to technical problems, it was then used rarely until the Odstock dropped foot stimulator (ODFS) was developed in the early 1990s. The ODFS is a single-channel neuromuscular stimulator that corrects dropped foot by stimulating the common peroneal nerve using self-adhesive skin surface electrodes placed on the side of the leg. The electrical stimulation causes dorsiflexion and eversion of the foot. When this is timed to the gait cycle using foot switches placed in the shoe, walking performance can be significantly improved.

Most studies of FES have looked at people with stroke. In two randomised controlled trials of FES to the leg after stroke, positive effects were seen both for spasticity and for walking ability.[55,56] Spasticity was assessed using the Wartenberg pendulum test[57] or a composite spasticity score.[56] Further small, mainly observational or single-case, studies of the application of FES to the leg have also been reported in patients with spinal cord injuries, head injuries or cerebral palsy, with promising results.[58,59]

FES can also be used for the arm, with positive results being seen in the stroke population for reduction in shoulder pain (perhaps mostly through reducing subluxation rather than spasticity) and improvements in motor recovery.[60–63]

FES and spasticity

The observation of a reduction in quadriceps tone in the randomised control trial of FES for foot drop in 32 stroke patients[55] is very interesting. Not only does stimulation of the common peroneal nerve result in dorsiflexion and eversion of the foot, but also, by triggering a flexion withdrawal reflex, knee and hip flexion occurs. The authors of this study hypothesise that such activity in the hamstrings may give rise to reciprocal inhibition in the quadriceps through Ia inhibitory neurones, and after much repetition neuroplastic changes could occur, resulting in reduced quadriceps tone.[57,64] Thus FES may impact on leg stiffness by reducing both the non-neural component (through repetitive ankle dorsiflexion increasing the length of the gastrocnemius and soleus muscles) and the neural aspect of spasticity (by reciprocal inhibition). Evidence to support this theory comes from the demonstration of a modest carryover effect of improvement in walking when not using the ODFS[64] and a sustained improvement over 3 months following upper-limb neurostimulation treatment post stroke.[63]

CONCLUSIONS

Attention to the physical management of spasticity is a vital component of any spasticity management plan.

Before a physical management programme can be instigated, a thorough assessment of the spasticity, its associated features and most importantly its impact on the individual is a necessity. The aims of the physical programme are to minimise non-neural stiffness and therefore contractures, while maintaining or improving the functional ability of the person.

Many different physical strategies are available, but very often a combination of these works best. However, the key to successful physical management lies in the individual understanding their spasticity and having the knowledge to incorporate an appropriate self-management programme into their daily life. It is therefore essential that, no matter what the level of function a person has, they have a suitable realistic programme that fits into their lifestyle with mechanisms for regular review to enable the physical intervention to change as the nature and degree of their spasticity change.

REFERENCES

1. Rizzo M, Hadjimichael O, Preiningerova J, Vollmer T. Prevelance and treatment of spasticity reported by multiple sclerosis patients. Mult Scler 2004;10:589–95.

2. Dietz V. Spastic movement disorder: What is the impact of research on clinical practice? J Neurol Neurosurg Psychiatry 2003;74:820–6.

3. Edwards S, Charlton PT. Splinting and the use of orthoses in the management of patients with neurological disorders. In: Edwards S (ed). Neurological Physiotherapy. A Problem Solving Approach. Edinburgh: Churchill Livingstone, 2002: 219–53.

4. Guttmann L. Comprehensive management and research. In: Guttmann L, Spinal Cord Injuries, 2nd edn. Oxford: Blackwell, 1976: 70–87.

5. Odeen I, Knutsson E. Evaluation of the effects of muscle stretch and weight load in patients with spastic paraplegia. Scand J Rehabil Med 1981;13:117–21.

6. Bohannon R, Larkin P. Passive ankle dorsiflexion increases in patients after a regimen of tilt table–wedge board standing. Phys Ther 1985:65:1676–8.

7. Bohannon R. Tilt table standing for reducing spasticity after spinal cord injury. Arch Phys Med Rehabil 1993;74:1121–2.

8. Kunkel C, Scremin E, Eisenberg B et al. Effect of 'standing' on spasticity, contracture, and osteoporosis in paralyzed males. Arch Phys Med Rehabil 1993;74:73–8.

9. Tremblay F, Malouin F, Richards CL, Dumas F. Effects of prolonged muscle stretch on reflex and voluntary muscle activations in children with spastic cerebral palsy. Scand J Rehabil Med 1990;22:171–80.

10. Tsai K, Yeh C, Chang H, Chen J. Effects of a single session of prolonged muscle stretch on spastic muscle of stroke patients. Proc Natl Sci Counc Repub China B 2001;25:76–81.

11. Multiple Sclerosis. NICE Guidelines, 2003.

12. Richardson DLA. The use of the tilt-table to affect passive tendo-achillis stretch in a patient with head injury. Physiother Theory Pract 1991;7:45–50.

13. Walter J, Soal P, Sacks J et al. Indications for a home standing programme for individuals with spinal cord injury. J Spinal Cord Med 1999;22:152–8.

14. Eng J, Levins S, Townson A et al. Use of prolonged standing for individuals with spinal cord injuries. Phys Ther 2001;81:1392–9.

15. Dunn R, Walter J, Lucero Y et al. Follow-up assessment of standing mobility device users. Asst Technol 1998;10:84–93.

16. Pope P. Management of the physical condition in patients with chronic and severe neurological pathologies. Physiotherapy 1992;78:896–903.

17. Gracies J. Pathophysiology of impairment in patients with spasticity and use of stretch as a treatment of spastic hypertonia. Phys Med Rehabil Clin North Am 2001;12:747–68.

18. Bruton A. Muscle plasticity: response to training and de-training. Physiotherapy 2002;88:398–408.

19. Dodd K, Taylor N, Damiano D. A systematic review of the effectiveness of strength-training programs for people with cerebral palsy. Arch Phys Med Rehabil 2002;83:1157–64.

20. Andersson C, Grooten W, Hellsten M et al. Adults with cerebral palsy: walking ability after progressive strength training. Develop Med Child Neurol 2003;45:220–8.

21. Van Peppen R, Kwakkel G, Wood-Dauphinee S et al. The impact of physical therapy on functional outcomes after stroke: What is the evidence? Clin Rehabil 2004;18:833–62.

22. White L, McCoy S, Castellano V et al. Resistance training improves strength and functional capacity in persons with multiple sclerosis. Mult Scler 2004;10:668–74.

23. Petajan JH, Gappmaier E, White A et al. Impact of aerobic training on fitness and quality of life as a

measure of rehabilitation outcome in patient with multiple sclerosis. Ann Neurol 1996;39:432–41.

24. O'Connell R. Exercise therapy in multiple sclerosis. Physiother Ireland 2005;26:23–6.

25. Rietberg M, Brooks D, Uitdehaag B, Kwakkel G. Exercise therapy for multiple sclerosis. Cochrane Database Syst Rev. 2004;(3):CD003980.

26. Schmit BD, Dewald JP, Rymer WZ. Stretch reflex adaptation in elbow flexors during repeated passive movements in unilateral brain-injured patients. Arch Phys Med Rehabil 2000;81:269–78.

27. Nuyens G, Weerdt W, Spaepen A et al. Reduction of spastic hypertonia during repeated passive knee movements in stroke patients. Arch Phys Med Rehabil 2002;83:930–5.

28. Kakebeeke T, Lechner H, Knapp P. The effects of passive cycling movements on spasticity after spinal cord injury: preliminary results. Spinal Cord 2005;43:483–8.

29. Rosche J, Paulus C, Maisch U et al. The effects of therapy on spasticity utilising a motorised exercise-cycle. Spinal Cord 1997;35:176–8.

30. O'Dwyer N, Ada L, Neilson P. Spasticity and muscle contracture following stroke. Brain 1996;119:1737–49.

31. Goldspink G, Tabary C, Tabary J et al. Effect of denervation on the adaptation of sarcomere number and muscle extensibility on the functional length of muscles. J Physiol 1974;236:733–42.

32. Williams PE. Use of intermittent stretch in the prevention of serial sarcomere loss in immobilised muscle. Ann Rheum Dis 1990;49:316–17.

33. Tardieu C, Lespargot C, Tabary C, Bret M. For how long must the soleus muscle be stretched each day to prevent contracture? Dev Med Child Neurol 1988;30:3–10.

34. Harvey L, Batty J, Crosbie J et al. A randomised trial assessing the effects of 4 weeks of daily stretching on ankle mobility in patients with spinal cord injuries. Arch Phys Med Rehabil 2000;81:1340–7.

35. Turton A, Britton E. A pilot randomised controlled trial of a daily muscle stretch routine to prevent contractures in the arm after stroke. Clin Rehabil 2005;19:600–12.

36. Akbyrak T, Armutlu K, Gunel N, Nurlu G. Assessment of the short term effect of antispastic positioning on spasticity. Paediatr Int 2005;47:440–5.

37. Odeen I. Reduction of muscular hypertonus by long-term muscle stretch. Scand J Rehabil Med 1981;13:93–9.

38. Kirkwood C, Bardsley G. Seating and positioning in spasticity. In: Barnes MP, Johnson GR (eds). Upper Motor Neurone Syndrome and Spasticity. Cambridge: Cambridge University Press, 2001:112–41.

39. Herman JH, Lange ML. Seating and positioning to manage spasticity after brain injury. Neurorehabilitation 1999;12:105–17.

40. Pope P. Posture management and special seating. In: Edwards S (ed). Neurological Physiotherapy. A Problem Solving Approach. Edinburgh: Churchill Livingstone, 2002:189–217.

41. Chan A, Heck C. The effects of tilting seat position of a wheelchair on respiration, posture, fatigue, voice volume and exertion: outcomes in individuals with advanced multiple sclerosis. J Rehabil Outcomes Meas 1999;3(4):1–14.

42. Rose G. Orthotics: Principles and Practice. London: Heinemann, 1986.

43. Association of Chartered Physiotherapists Interested in Neurology. Clinical Practice Guidelines on Splinting Adults with Neurological Dysfunction. Chartered Society of Physiotherapy, 1998.

44. Mortenson P, Eng J. The use of casts in the management of joint mobility and hypertonia following brain injury in adults: a systematic review. Phys Ther 2003;83:648–58.

45. Verplancke D, Snape S, Salisbury C, Ward A. A randomised controlled trial of botulinum toxin on lower limb spasticity following acute acquired severe brain injury. Clin Rehabil 2005;19:117–25.

46. Lannin N, Horsley S, Herbert R et al. Splinting the hand in the functional position after brain impairment: a randomised controlled trial. Arch Phys Med Rehabil 2003;84:297–302.

47. Lannin N, Herbert R. Is hand splinting effective for adults following stroke? A systematic review and methodological critique of published research. Clin Rehabil 2003;17:807–16.

48. Gracies J, Marosszeky J, Renton R et al. Short term effects of dynamic lycra splints on upper limb in hemiplegic patients. Arch Phys Med Rehabil 2000;81:1547–55.

49. Iwata M, Kondo I, Sato Y et al. An ankle foot orthosis with inhibitor bar: effect on gait. Arch Phys Med Rehabil 2003;84:924–7.

50. Kent R, Gilbertson L, Geddes J. Orthotic devices for abnormal limb posture after stroke or non-progressive cerebral causes of spasticity. Cochrane Database Syst Rev 2001;(4):CD003694.

51. Royal College of Physicians (RCP) Guidelines for the use of Botulinum Toxin (BTX) in the Management of Adult Spacticity. PUB 15113 020.

52. Mackay S, Wallen M. Re-examining the effects of the soft splint on acute hypertonicity at the elbow. Austr Occup Ther J 1996;43:51–9.

53. Kesiktas N, Paker N, Erdogan N et al. The use of hydrotherapy for the management of spacticity. Am Soc Neurorehabil 2004;18:269–73.

54. Liberson W, Holmquest H, Scott M. Functional electrotherapy: stimulation of the common peroneal nerve synchronised with the swing phase of gait of hemiplegic subjects. Arch Phys Med Rehabil 1961;42:202–5.

55. Burridge J, Taylor P, Hagan S et al. The effects of common peroneal stimulation on the effort and speed of walking: a randomised controlled clinical trial with chronic hemiplegic patients. Clin Rehabil 1997;11:201–10.

56. Yan T, Hui-Chan CW, Li LS. Functional electrical stimulation improves motor recovery of the lower extremity and walking ability of subjects with first acute stroke: a randomised placebo-controlled trial. Stroke 2005;36:80–5.

57. Burridge J, Taylor P, Hagan SA et al. The effect on the spasticity of the quadriceps muscles of stimulation of the common peroneal nerve of chronic hemiplegic subjects during walking. Physiotherapy 1997;83:82–9.

58. Granat MH, Ferguson AC, Andrews BJ, Delargy M. The role of functional electrical stimulation in the rehabilitation of patients with incomplete spinal cord injury- observed benefit during gait studies. Paraplegia 1993;31:207–15.

59. Kralj A, Acimovic R, Stanic U. Enhancement of hemiplegic patient rehabilitation by means of functional electrical stimulation. Prosthet Orthot Int 1993;17:107–14.

60. Chae J, Yu DT, Walker ME et al. Intramuscular electrical stimulation for hemiplegic shoulder pain: a 12-month follow-up of a multiple-center, randomised clinical trial. Am J Phys Med Rehabil 2005;84:832–42.

61. Price CI, Pandyan AD. Electrical stimulation for preventing and treating post-stroke shoulder pain: a systematic Cochrane Review. Clin Rehabil 2001;15:5–19.

62. Glanz M, Klawansky S, Stason W et al. Functional electrostimulation in poststroke rehabilitation: a meta-analysis of the randomised controlled trials. Arch Phys Med Rehabil 1996;77:549–53.

63. Chae J, Bethoux F, Bohine T et al. Neuromuscular stimulation for upper extremity motor and functional recovery in acute hemiplegia. Stroke 1998;29:975–9.

64. Taylor PN, Burridge JH, Dunkerley AL et al. Clinical use of the Odstock dropped foot stimulator: its effect on the speed and effort of walking. Arch Phys Med Rehabil 1999;80:1577–83.

Chapter 5

Oral medication

Valerie L Stevenson

There is no agreed evidence-based model available for the systematic pharmacological management of spasticity, and much of what is done is based on a logical and pragmatic approach. The use of drugs should of course always be an adjunct to good general management, with an emphasis on ongoing education of all involved, including the individual, family members, carers and health professionals. Providing an information sheet to complement verbal information can be extremely helpful in putting oral medication in the context of effective general spasticity management (Appendix 3). Continuity of care, combined with documentation of the evolving impact of spasticity, is necessary to enable ongoing assessment of change and to aid in the appropriate choice and timing of any pharmacological intervention. Knowledge of the trigger and aggravating factors detailed in Chapter 3 is particularly important, as they can exacerbate spasticity and its associated features. Far too often, pharmacological treatment is escalated before appropriate strategies to manage bladder and bowel function, skin integrity, soft tissue length and positioning are instigated. Attention to these simple but essential areas is paramount at all stages of management, and will ensure that drugs are used at appropriate times and dosages.

Drug treatment can be used for generalised spasticity, targeted to focal problems for example with the use of botulinum toxin or chemical neurolysis (Chapter 6), or regionally with intrathecal baclofen or phenol (Chapter 7). This chapter will cover the orally administered drugs commonly used for spasticity and will discuss their modes of action, side-effect profiles, dosage schedules and evidence base.

GENERAL ISSUES WHEN PRESCRIBING ORAL MEDICATION

Once the decision has been made to start medication to help with spasticity management, it is important to focus on the aims of treatment. These should be based on improving function or relieving troublesome symptoms rather than simply reducing the degree of spasticity. The identification of such treatment goals will help optimise drug therapy not only in terms of choice of agent but also in timing and dose. For example, painful nocturnal spasms may best be managed with a long-acting agent taken at night-time that has sedative side-effects. Alternatively, stiffness and spasms, which interfere with a person's morning transfers and personal care, may benefit from medication taken on waking prior to the person transferring out of bed. Dosages for individuals who are walking, and who may be relying on their spasticity to do so, are often lower than in those who use a wheelchair for mobility.

A general rule with all medication is to 'start low and go slow'. It may therefore take some time to optimise a treatment regime, but this approach will limit any deleterious effects on function or unwanted side-effects. When trialling a drug, it may take several weeks to increase to a level that is effective without precipitating side-effects due to a too-rapid escalation. It is therefore important that drugs are not 'discarded' before the dose reaches the maximum level or side-effects occur.

Unfortunately, all currently available drug treatments for spasticity can have side-effects, the most common of which are drowsiness and weakness. It is therefore extremely important to ensure that the individual is on the lowest dose regime that effectively controls their symptoms. The most common reported side-effect is of increased weakness, although it is of course important to recognise that this may actually be as a result of unmasking the degree of underlying weakness by reducing tone (spasticity) that was functionally useful.

Taking an effective drug history is essential

Often individuals with troublesome spasticity report that they have tried 'everything' and nothing works. However, once a careful drug history has been obtained detailing each drug, when it was trialled, how long for and at what dose, it is often apparent that although all of the commonly used agents have been tried, these were often at a level that was too low, too high or for too short a time. Paradoxically, drugs may be discarded due to side-effects of weakness or floppiness, which are actually evidence that the drug worked but was perhaps prescribed at too high a dose for the individual, or taken at inappropriate times.

It is therefore essential that when a drug is trialled, it be started at a low dose and gradually increased according to efficacy either up to a level where side-effects occur or up to the maximum dose. If side-effects do occur, it is worth pausing for a short time at a level that is tolerated before retrying the dose escalation. Sometimes, despite titrating a drug up to the maximum level, adding a second agent as combination therapy is necessary to control symptoms.

Combination drug regimes

Despite optimal nursing, physiotherapy input and the use of physical adjuncts such as specialist seating systems, it is not always possible to control spasticity with a single drug without causing unacceptable side-effects. It is therefore preferable to treat an individual with a combination of agents at lower doses to enable effective treatment within the realm of tolerable side-

effects. It is of course also possible to combine oral therapy with local or regional treatments as outlined in the following chapters.

All of the commonly used drugs – baclofen, tizanidine, benzodiazepines, dantrolene and gabapentin – can be used alone as monotherapy or in combination with each other. Which combination to use may be based on the presence of associated features or by considering their modes of action. For example, if neuropathic pain is problematic as well as spasticity, gabapentin may be the most appropriate first-line add-on agent, whereas dantrolene (the only drug that acts directly on skeletal muscle) can be a useful adjunct to the other centrally acting agents.

There is no right or wrong way to titrate drugs in combination, and understandably both health professionals and the individuals concerned are keen to avoid polypharmacy. As a general rule, if the first-line drug proves to be partially effective but causes side-effects at higher doses then it can be maintained at the highest level the individual can tolerate comfortably, with the second-line drug being added in and titrated upwards. If spasticity becomes well managed on this regime, the first drug can be cautiously withdrawn to see if monotherapy with the second-line drug alone is sufficient to achieve the goal of treatment. Likewise, if necessary, a third drug can be introduced along the same principles. If a drug is trialled that is completely ineffective either as a first-line treatment or as an adjunct, it can be gradually withdrawn before the next agent is tried.

Optimising the effects of drug regimes

Many individuals take medications in a rather haphazard fashion through choice due to concerns over side-effects, because of difficulties administering medications or due to other issues such as cognitive difficulties impacting on their ability to remember to take complicated dosage regimes. Missing doses or taking medication at inappropriate times can clearly impact on the efficacy of drug regimes: several strategies to aid individuals to optimally manage their medication can then be employed (Table 5.1).

Monitoring the effects of medication

Once individuals commence medication for their spasticity, it is of course essential that the effects of this be carefully monitored. This needs to be a team

Table 5.1 Mechanisms to aid in optimising drug treatments for spasticity

Provision of written information

Information on the actions and side-effects of commonly used drugs in the context of general management of spasticity (triggers and aggravating factors, stretches, exercises and posture). See Appendix 3

Identification of clear treatment goals

This will aid in the choice of agent (e.g. a drug with sedative side-effects to aid in nocturnal spasms), the timing of the drug regime and the dose, according to goal achievement

Use of appropriate aids

The use of a dossette box with or without a pager/timer device can help ensure that medication is taken accurately and at appropriate times

Appropriate formulation

Consider the use of liquid preparations if available, which are easier to swallow and can be administered via a nasogastric or gastrostomy tube

Mechanism for review of efficacy and side-effects

There is a clear responsibility for professionals to monitor efficacy: this may be best done by community teams or district nurses. A mechanism should be in place for individuals to feedback effects of drugs to the team

responsibility, including the individual with spasticity. Observations of any difficulties or improvements with everyday tasks such as washing and dressing are extremely valuable. Carers or district nurses, if applicable, may be the individuals with the most day-to-day knowledge, and should be encouraged to take an active role in monitoring the effectiveness of drug regimes. During titration phases, the physiotherapist is able to give a clear objective assessment on the effects of medication changes, which will help guide future treatment. Although the neurologist or rehabilitation physician may be responsible for prescribing or guiding therapy, the actual titration dosage will often be under the direct control of the General Practitioner, and it is therefore essential that the whole team communicate effectively with each other across both primary and secondary care. The routine practice of copying all correspondence to patients is one example where communication links have been greatly improved over recent years.[1]

ORAL MEDICATION FOR SPASTICITY

Prescribing details for all of the commonly used drugs, as well as some recently trialled agents, will be discussed in detail here; those frequently utilised are summarised in Table 5.2.

Baclofen

This is the most commonly used drug for spasticity of both cerebral and spinal origin. It is usually given orally as either a tablet or a liquid preparation; however, it can also be used intrathecally (Chapter 7).

Mode of action

The precise mechanisms of action of baclofen are not fully understood; however, the predominant effect appears to be inhibition of both monosynaptic and polysynaptic reflexes at the spinal level, although actions at supraspinal sites may also contribute to its clinical effect.

Baclofen is an analogue of the inhibitory neurotransmitter γ-aminobutyric acid (GABA) and binds to $GABA_B$ receptors, which are found predominantly presynaptically in the Ia sensory afferent neurones, the interneurones and also postsynaptically in the motor neurones.[2,3] The presynaptic agonistic action on $GABA_B$ receptors reduces calcium influx and suppresses the release of excitatory neurotransmitters, including glutamate. In addition, there is a postsynaptic increase in potassium conductance, the net result of these actions being inhibition of both monosynaptic and polysynaptic reflexes.[4–6]

Evidence base

Most of the clinical trials of baclofen in the management of spasticity have involved patients with either multiple sclerosis (MS) or spinal cord injury. Few have concentrated on spasticity of cerebral origin, including stroke or traumatic brain injury. Although most have shown a positive effect of baclofen in reducing hypertonia and spasms, little attention has been paid to functional benefit.[7]

The first placebo-controlled trials of baclofen were performed in the 1970s. Studies in spinal cord injury showed a reduction in spasticity, less frequent spasms and also beneficial effects on bladder control.[8,9]

In a small crossover study of children with cerebral palsy, baclofen was shown to reduce the Ashworth

Table 5.2 The commonly used oral drugs for spasticity

Drug	Starting dose	Maximum dose	Side-effects
Baclofen	5–10 mg daily	120 mg daily, usually in 3 divided doses	Drowsiness, weakness, paraesthesiae, nausea, vomiting
Tizanidine	2 mg daily	36 mg daily, usually in 3 or 4 divided doses	Drowsiness, weakness, dry mouth, postural hypotension • *Monitor liver function*
Dantrolene	25 mg daily	400 mg daily, usually in 4 divided doses	Anorexia, nausea, vomiting, drowsiness, weakness, dizziness, paraesthesiae • *Monitor liver function*
Diazepam	2 mg daily	40–60 mg daily, usually in 3 or 4 divided doses	Drowsiness, reduced attention, memory impairment • *Dependency and withdrawal syndromes*
Clonazepam	0.25–0.5 mg, usually at night-time	3mg, usually in 3 divided doses	Same as diazepam
Gabapentin	300 mg daily (can start at 100 mg daily)	2400 mg daily, usually in 3 divided doses	Drowsiness, somnolence, dizziness

score compared with placebo, but no difference was noted on 'overall evaluation'.[10]

A placebo-controlled trial in stroke also showed a beneficial effect on the Ashworth score, but no change in the incapacity status scale. Overall evaluation was, however, significantly different between the treated and placebo groups.[11] No difference in efficacy or tolerability was seen in a comparison study between baclofen and tizanidine in a stroke population.[12]

Baclofen has been evaluated in several studies in MS.[13–15] Most showed a significant change in the Ashworth score, with reduced spasms and increased range of motion reported; none of the studies reported any effect on function. Three of the MS studies compared baclofen with diazepam, with no significant difference in effect, but generally patients preferred baclofen due to its reduced side-effect profile.[16–18]

Side-effects

Side-effects during baclofen treatment may be troublesome and are reported to affect up to 45% of users;[19] they may be a particular problem in the elderly or those with spasticity of cerebral origin who have additional cognitive impairment. Reducing the dose slightly or slowing the rate of dose titration can, however, often moderate them. The most frequently reported effects in clinical trials have been sedation, drowsiness, weakness, paraesthesiae, nausea, vomiting and dry mouth.[14] Other reported effects have included psychosis and dyskinesias.[20,21]

It is important to note that baclofen should be used with caution in individuals with a history of convulsions, as the seizure threshold may be reduced, with possible loss of control of their epilepsy.

Sudden withdrawal should be avoided in all individuals, as it may precipitate seizures, confusion, anxiety and hallucinations.[22]

Pharmacokinetics and dosage regime

Baclofen is rapidly absorbed through the gastrointestinal tract, so its effects can be appreciated quickly; peak plasma levels can occur as soon as 1 hour. It is therefore a useful strategy to administer baclofen half an hour before the clinical effects are particularly wanted, for example getting out of bed in the morning.

The half-life of baclofen is of the order of 3–4 hours, so often a three times daily regime is necessary to maintain clinical effectiveness throughout the whole day.

The recommended dose range is up to 120 mg daily, although higher doses have been reported for use in MS.[23] Tolerance may be an issue at higher doses due to side-effects. Baclofen is predominantly excreted by the kidneys: therefore it may be necessary to reduce the dose in individuals with renal impairment.

The usual starting dose of baclofen is 5–10 mg daily; it can then be gradually titrated upwards according to effect and tolerance. If side-effects occur, it may be necessary to reduce the dosage or slow down the titration. If no benefit is seen at 120 mg daily or the maximum tolerated dose then the baclofen should be reduced gradually and withdrawn, remembering that it should never be abruptly stopped due to the risk of withdrawal seizures.[22]

Tizanidine

Tizanidine was licensed for the management of spasticity in the 1990s. As it has a different mechanism of action to baclofen, it can sometimes be used to good effect in combination with the latter if monotherapy with either drug is insufficient.

Mode of action

Like baclofen, the precise mechanisms of action of tizanidine are not fully understood. It is however known that it acts as a potent selective α_2-adrenergic receptor agonist throughout the central nervous system (CNS), although the major effect is on spinal polysynaptic reflexes. Through both direct impairment of excitatory amino acid (glutamate and aspartate) release from spinal interneurones and a concomitant inhibition of facilitatory coeruleospinal pathways, there is a reduction in presynaptic excitatory interneuronal activity.[24] The clinical effects are a reduction of both tonic and phasic stretch reflexes as well as a reduction of co-contraction.[25]

Evidence base

Most of the reported studies have involved people with MS: these trials have been extensively reviewed.[13–15] In comparison with placebo, tizanidine has been shown to reduce muscle tone, frequency of spasms and clonus; no functional benefit has, however, been demonstrated. In comparison studies with diazepam, baclofen and tetrazepam, all four drugs appear to be of equal efficacy, although tizanidine had fewer side-effects than diazepam, but was comparable to baclofen.

In a study of 124 patients with spinal cord injury, tizanidine was found to significantly reduce spasticity and spasms compared with placebo, but no changes in functional assessment were seen.[26]

Two studies in stroke revealed a reduction in tone and spasms compared with placebo[27] and equal efficacy to baclofen.[12]

Side-effects

Tizanidine is generally well tolerated. In trials comparing tizanidine with baclofen in MS, the incidence and severity of side-effects were broadly similar.[14] The most commonly reported side-effects are sedation, drowsiness, weakness, dry mouth and postural hypotension. Interestingly, although comparative studies between baclofen and tizanidine have suggested a slight preference by patients and investigators for baclofen, the same trials reported slightly more weakness as a side-effect with baclofen than with tizanidine.[13]

Changes in liver function tests have been documented in subjects taking tizanidine, and rare cases of acute fulminant hepatitis have been reported. It is therefore recommended that individuals have their liver function tested before commencement of therapy and then at 2 weeks, 1 month, 3 months and 6 months after, while therapy is stabilised.

Pharmacokinetics and dosage regime

Tizanidine, like baclofen, is also rapidly absorbed through the gastrointestinal tract, with peak plasma levels occurring at 1–2 hours. The half-life is of the order of 2–4 hours, so a three or even four times daily regime may be appropriate for individuals. Tizanidine is usually started at a dose of 2 mg daily, with increments every few days to a maximum of 36 mg daily. As previously outlined, it is necessary to check liver function before initiating treatment and then to undertake regular monitoring during dose titration and for the first few months of treatment. Tolerance may be an issue at higher doses due to side-effects, particularly sedation. As with other agents, if side-effects occur, it may be necessary to reduce the dosage, divide the total daily dose further or slow down the titration.

Dantrolene

Dantrolene is a novel drug for spasticity management, as it is the only available agent that works outside the CNS, with a direct action on skeletal muscle. It is therefore applicable to spasticity originating from both spinal and supraspinal lesions and is a useful adjunct to a centrally acting agent for combination therapy.

Mode of action

Dantrolene acts through decreasing the excitation coupling reaction within skeletal muscle fibres; this is achieved by suppression of calcium ion release from the sarcoplasmic reticulum.[28–30] Its greatest effect is on the force of contraction in fast-twitch fibres at low rates of neural stimulation and at shorter muscle lengths.[31] Additionally, there appears to be a dose-dependent reduction in activity of phasic stretch reflexes more than tonic ones, suggesting that dantrolene may be particularly useful for control of spasms.[29] Dantrolene is known to have an effect on both intra- and extrafusal fibres, suggesting that it may also alter spindle sensitivity (Chapter 1), which could account for some of its anti-spasticity effect.[5]

Evidence base

When compared with placebo in the MS population, dantrolene appears to produce an improvement in spasticity and spasms; however, none of the trials used validated outcome measures and several were unblinded.[13,14] In a crossover study comparing dantrolene with diazepam, both drugs reduced spasticity and spasms, although both were associated with significant side-effects; 22 of the 42 patients who completed the study preferred dantrolene, 13 preferred diazepam and 7 neither drug.[32]

Moderate beneficial effects have also been shown in spinal cord injury,[33] stroke[34,35] and cerebral palsy.[36] Again, none of the trials demonstrated any change in function.

Side-effects

Unfortunately, side-effects are fairly frequent with dantrolene, although they may ameliorate with time; however, the risk of hepatotoxicity is the major limiting factor to its use.

The most commonly reported side-effects are gastrointestinal symptoms of anorexia, nausea, vomiting and diarrhoea. Additionally, there may be some CNS effects of drowsiness, fatigue, weakness, dizziness and paraesthesiae. Although weakness has been reported, maximum voluntary muscle power has been assessed as being reduced to only 93%.[37]

Acute hepatitis, which may be fatal, is recognised as an idiosyncratic reaction to dantrolene, and therefore, like tizanidine, liver function tests are mandatory before initiating therapy and regularly while on treatment. The risk of fatal hepatonecrosis is increased in women, those on larger doses (> 300 mg/day) or on long-term treatment (> 60 days), and those taking concomitant drugs also metabolised in the liver, such as oestrogens.[28,30]

Pharmacokinetics and dosage regime

Dantrolene is absorbed in the small intestine and metabolised in the liver to its active metabolite 5-hydroxydantrolene. Peak plasma levels occur at 3–6 hours for the inactive drug and 4–8 hours for the active metabolite. The half-life is of the order of 15 hours.[5]

Treatment regimes are usually started at a dose of 25 mg once daily and increased gradually by 25 mg increments every few days to a maximum of 100 mg four times a day. The divided dosage regime helps to limit gastrointestinal side-effects.

As already outlined, it is necessary to check liver function before initiating treatment and then regularly throughout treatment.

Benzodiazepines

Benzodiazepines were the first class of drugs used to treat spasticity, and diazepam specifically has a long history of use, particularly in spasticity of spinal origin.[38,39] The main limitation to their use in current therapeutic regimes is the side-effect profile.

Diazepam, chlordiazepoxide and clonazepam are long-acting agents, whereas lorazepam, oxazepam and alprazolam are shorter-acting. The two most commonly prescribed benzodiazepines for spasticity are the longer-acting agents diazepam and clonazepam.

Mode of action

Like baclofen, the effect of benzodiazepines is through modulation of GABAergic transmission;

however, they exert their influence via stimulation of $GABA_A$ receptors, unlike baclofen, which acts on $GABA_B$ receptors. $GABA_A$ receptors are coupled to a chloride ionosphere complex, and once binding occurs to the receptors, the chloride ion channels are opened, allowing the postsynaptic effects of GABA to be realised, with a reduction in both mono- and polysynaptic spinal reflexes.[40–42]

Evidence base

The efficacy of diazepam in spinal cord injury has been proven in two crossover trials.[38,39] In cerebral palsy, it has also been noted to be beneficial for athetosis as well as spasticity.[43,44]

In MS, the trials have mostly been comparative studies with other agents (baclofen, tizanidine and ketazolam); these studies have shown similar efficacy between diazepam and the other drugs, but there was an excess of side-effects in the diazepam-treated groups.[14]

Side-effects

These are frequent and can be divided into CNS depressant effects, toxicity and withdrawal syndromes. Most commonly seen are the depressant effects of drowsiness, sedation, reduced attention and memory impairment. Cognitive changes may be marked in the elderly or in those with organic brain disease.

Occasionally, toxic symptoms of ataxia, vertigo, headache, gastrointestinal symptoms, behavioural disturbance, hypotension and coma can occur.

Physiological dependence can also occur, with an associated withdrawal syndrome. Benzodiazepines should always be reduced slowly and abrupt cessation of therapy avoided. Withdrawal symptoms include anxiety, agitation, restlessness, irritability, tremor, muscle twitching, seizures, psychosis and even death. The intensity of withdrawal symptoms is related to the dose and duration of treatment. Even when benzodiazepines are withdrawn slowly, such symptoms may persist for 6 months.[5,45]

Pharmacokinetics and dosage regime

Diazepam is rapidly absorbed, with peak plasma levels being reached in about 1 hour. It is metabolised in the liver to the active components N-desmethyldiazepam and oxazepam, both of which are protein-bound. The half-life is variable and long (20–80 hours). Individuals with low-albumin states or hepatic impairment may be predisposed to side-effects or toxicity with any of the benzodiazepines.

Diazepam is usually started at a dose of 2 mg once or twice daily, and can be titrated up to 40–60 mg/day in three or four divided doses. However, side-effects often limit daytime use.

Due to the commonest side-effect of sedation, benzodiazepines are often preferred for night-time use only. Clonazepam appears to be particularly useful for nocturnal spasms and stiffness; it can be started at a dose of 0.25–0.5 mg at night. Dose escalation of clonazepam above 1 mg three times a day is rarely tolerated.

Gabapentin

This is the newest addition to the range of drugs routinely prescribed to relieve spasticity. It was initially launched as an anticonvulsant for partial seizures in the early 1990s, but its main use over recent years has been due to its effects on neuropathic pain. Following some recent small studies, it has also gained favour as an anti-spasticity agent, where it appears to be a useful adjunct, which is on the whole well tolerated.

Mode of action

Like baclofen and benzodiazepines, gabapentin is another GABAergic drug; however, it does not bind with either $GABA_A$ or $GABA_B$ receptors.

Its specific mode of action is unknown, but it has been shown to bind to the $\alpha 2\delta$ subunit of calcium channels, and thus it may modulate cell function through alterations in calcium ion influx.[46] In addition, gabapentin appears to reduce the release of several monoamine neurotransmitters, including glutamate, while increasing GABA synthesis.[47,48]

Evidence base

Four small double-blind, placebo-controlled randomised studies have been performed to date. Two of these were in MS patients,[49,50] one was in spinal cord injury alone[51] and another included patients with any cause of upper motor neurone (UMN) syndrome.[52] All showed a beneficial effect of gabapentin on measures of spasticity; tolerability also appeared favourable.

Side-effects

Generally, gabapentin is well tolerated. Its main adverse effects are drowsiness, somnolence and dizziness. The dosage regime does allow for a fairly rapid dose titration; however, if side-effects occur, this can be slowed down or the total dose reduced.

There are no significant drug–drug interactions and no necessity to perform blood monitoring.

Pharmacokinetics and dosage regime

Gabapentin has an attractive pharmacokinetic profile. It is absorbed by an active and saturable transport system, and has a high volume of distribution. Gabapentin is not bound to plasma proteins, does not induce hepatic enzymes and is not metabolised; it is excreted unchanged by the kidneys. The half-life is of the order of 6–8 hours.[53]

Normal dosage regimes are three times daily. The normal starting dose is 300 mg once a day (although this can be reduced to 100 mg daily in susceptible individuals), increasing to 300 mg twice a day and then 300 mg three times a day. Further increments of 300–600 mg can then be made every few days up to a total daily dose of 2400 mg.

Cannabinoids

Cannabis has been used recreationally for many hundreds of years, and there is evidence of its medicinal use in Europe dating back to the 13th century.[54] More recently, it has been advocated for pain relief and spasticity by individuals who have experienced spinal cord injuries, and has particularly gained favour within the MS population. Cannabis in its natural form is classified as a class C drug in the UK; its possession and supply remain illegal.

The main active ingredient of the cannabis plant (*Cannabis sativa*) is Δ^9-tetrahydrocannabinol (THC), which is available as a synthetic pharmaceutical product (Marinol). As THC is only one of over 60 cannabinoids, it is of course possible that its action is influenced by the presence of other cannabinoids. For this reason, studies have focused not only on the effectiveness of THC but also on that of whole plant extracts (available in the UK as an oromucosal spray: Sativex).

Mode of action

Cannabinoids exert their effect through receptors, two of which have been isolated. The CB2 receptors are expressed predominantly by leucocytes and do not appear to have any neurological activity. CNS effects are mediated via CB1 receptors and possibly by further as-yet unknown receptors. CB1 is expressed strongly in the cerebellum, hippocampus and basal ganglia, which explains the predominant effect of cannabinoids on short-term memory and coordination.[55] However, there are also high concentrations of CB1 in the dorsal primary afferent spinal cord regions, where cannabinoids may have their effects on pain and possibly spasticity.

The main function of the CB1 endocannabinoid system is in the regulation of synaptic neurotransmission of both excitatory and inhibitory pathways. Most neurotransmitters appear to be susceptible to these effects, but the exact mechanisms are yet to be elucidated.[55,56]

Evidence base

Cannabis has been used by individuals with MS for many years on the basis of anecdotal evidence and on the results of several mostly small studies, which have suggested subjective improvement in symptoms but no objective changes. Benefits in self-reported assessments of pain, spasms, sleeping, bladder control and spasticity have been demonstrated.[57–63]

Two large studies have recently been completed from which it was hoped clinical effectiveness would be clarified. The first was a trial of 630 subjects randomised to oral placebo, THC or cannabis extract.[59] There was no effect in the primary outcome measure of a change in Ashworth score over the 13-week treatment period. Improvement was seen on patient-reported category rating scales for pain, sleep quality, spasms and spasticity; however, this was in the context of a degree of patient unmasking in the active treatment groups. It is possible that a significant effect on the Ashworth score could have been achieved at higher doses, but most subjects did not reach their target doses due to unacceptable side-effects. The conclusion from this study was that although no major effect on spasticity was noted, some evidence was provided on symptom relief that deserves further attention.[59] Following on from this study, participants were invited to continue study medication (or placebo) in a blinded fashion for up to 1 year. Intention-to-treat analysis at 12 months revealed a significant beneficial effect on the Ashworth scores of the group receiving THC, but not those receiving cannabis extract.[64]

The second study involved 160 patients who were randomised to either a placebo sublingual spray or a cannabis extract spray. Patients recorded a 'primary symptom score' before and after treatment; this was a visual analogue score of their worst symptom from a choice of five (spasticity, spasms, pain, bladder dysfunction or tremor). There was no significant difference in these scores between treatment and placebo; however, in the spasticity subset, there was a significant treatment effect. No difference was seen in Ashworth scores. As in the first study, there was a considerable placebo effect.[58]

The evidence from these studies supports a symptomatic benefit for cannabinoids, as well as showing an objective improvement in spasticity as measured by the Ashworth scale for THC-treated individuals in the extended phase of the CAMS study.[64] This gives further support for a long-term study in MS to assess both symptomatic benefit and measures of disease progression.

Side-effects

The acute side-effects of cannabis are well known. It causes a psychoactive, mildly euphoric state, with some psychomotor slowing and cognitive changes particularly impacting on short-term memory. Anxiety, panic, paranoia and occasional psychosis can also occur. Other effects include appetite stimulation, hypotension, redness of the eyes, dry mouth and dizziness.

Concerns remain over long-term use and the possibility of cognitive impairment and an increased risk of psychosis.

Pharmacokinetics and dosage regime

The route of administration for pharmaceutical cannabis plant extract or cannabinoids is an important issue. Oral administration is the least efficient mode due to sequestration into fat and then slow and variable rates of release back into plasma.[65] There is also a significant degree of first-pass metabolism in the liver, causing problems with appropriate dosage levels and side-effects. Smoking, the traditional form

of delivery for cannabis, is of course not an option, as it has significant risks of lung cancer and other respiratory dysfunction.[66] Sublingual sprays, metered-dose inhalers and transdermal patch delivery systems are being proposed as alternative delivery options.[54]

Synthetic cannabinoids or pharmaceutical cannabis plant extract are not currently licensed for the management of spasticity in the UK, although Sativex is available on a named-patient basis.

Other oral agents

Many different drugs have been considered as possible anti-spasticity agents. Most have similar mechanisms of action as those already discussed; some have unacceptable side-effect profiles. None have been tested in appropriately designed studies, with the only evidence available being from open-label studies or anecdotal case reports.

Clonidine, like tizanidine, is an imidazaline derivative that acts at the α_2-adrenergic receptors. Its major use has been as an anti-hypertensive agent, but in a small study of individuals with spinal cord injury it was found to be beneficial for spasticity.[67] It is also available as a transdermal patch, which has been advocated for use in spinal spasticity with a preferential side-effect profile.[68] Its use is limited by hypotension and bradycardia.

Levetiracetam is a second-generation anticonvulsant drug whose mode of action is also incompletely understood. It is thought to promote inhibitory neurotransmission via modulation of $GABA_A$ and glycine receptors, and to depress high-voltage-activated calcium channels. In a small open-label series of 12 patients, a reduction in the Penn spasm score was seen following treatment with levetiracetam.[69]

Vigabatrin is a further anticonvulsant drug, whose use has been curtailed to infantile spasms due to the serious adverse effect observed on visual function. Despite some suggestions that it may ameliorate spasticity, it is unlikely to be of clinical benefit due to potential visual field constriction.[70]

Fampridine (sustained-release 4-aminopyridine) has been suggested to be helpful in patients with spinal cord injuries. It has also been advocated for relief of fatigue in MS, but its use has been limited by side-effects, including dizziness, paraesthesiae and seizures.[71]

Other agents that have been tried over the years include cyproheptadine, L-threonine, piracetam, progabide, riluzole, lamotrigine, thymoxamine, orphenadrine, phenothiazines, magnesium, memantine and glycine. No evidence exists for their beneficial effect on spasticity.[5,14,15,25,72]

CONCLUSIONS

Although oral medications have been in use for spasticity for over 50 years, the evidence that they have a positive impact on functional ability for the individual is generally lacking. Nevertheless, it appears clear that, when used in the appropriate setting of a management plan that incorporates all of the aspects essential for a coordinated multidisciplinary approach to spasticity management, they are a useful adjunct to physical measures. Education of the individual with spasticity about the commonly used drugs and their side-effects will help in monitoring the effect of medication and aid in optimising treatment regimes; this can be facilitated by providing an information sheet to patients and, if appropriate, carers or family members (Appendix 3).

Identification of clear treatment goals will guide the choice of agent as well as optimising the effect through appropriate advice on dose and timing. In addition, active, effective communication of these plans is paramount to the ongoing appropriate use of oral medication and, in the case of tizanidine or dantrolene, for essential blood monitoring.

All drugs can cause side-effects; however, with a systematic approach, these can usually be minimised by appropriate dosage regimes and titrations. The 'start low and go slow' rule should avoid most unpleasant side-effects.

REFERENCES

1. Department of Health. Copying Letters to Patients: Good Practice Guidelines. London: DoH, 2003.

2. Hill DR, Bowery NG. ³H-baclofen and ³H-GABA bind to bicuculline insensitive GABA-B sites in rat brain. Nature 1981;290:149–52.

3. Price GW, Kelly JS, Bowery NG. The location of GABA-B receptor binding sites in mammalian spinal cord. Synapse 1987;1:530–8.

4. Davies J. Selective depression of synaptic excitation in cat spinal neurons by baclofen: An inotophorectic study. Br J Pharm 1981;72:373–84.

5. Gracies JM, Elovic E, McGuire J, Simpson D. Traditional pharmacological treatments for spasticity. Part II: General and regional treatments. Muscle Nerve Suppl 1997;6:S92–120.

6. Nicoll RA. My close encounter with GABA(B) receptors. Biochem Pharmacol 2004;688:1667–74.

7. Montane E, Vallano A, Laporte JR. Oral antispastic drugs in nonprogressive neurologic diseases: a systematic review. Neurology 2004;63:1357–63.

8. Pinto OD, Polikar M, Debono G. Results of international clinical trials with Lioresal. Postgrad Med J 1972;48(Suppl 5):18–23.

9. Duncan GW, Shahani BT, Young RR. An evaluation of baclofen treatment for certain symptoms in patients with spinal cord lesions: a double blind cross over study. Neurology 1976;26:441–6.

10. Milla PJ, Jackson ADM. A controlled trial of baclofen in children with cerebral palsy. J Int Med Res 1997;5:398–404.

11. Medaer R, Hellebuyk H, Van Den Brande E et al. Treatment of spasticity due to stroke. A double-blind, cross-over trial comparing baclofen with placebo. Acta Therapeutica 1991;17:323–31.

12. Medici M, Pebet M, Ciblis D. A double-blind, long-term study of tizanidine ('Sirdalud') in spasticity due to cerebrovascular lesions. Curr Med Res Opin 1989;11:398–407.

13. Shakespeare DT, Boggild M, Young C. Anti-spasticity agents for multiple sclerosis. Cochrane Database Syst Rev 2003;(4):CD001332.

14. Beard S, Hunn A, Wight J. Treatments for spasticity and pain in multiple sclerosis: a systematic review. Health Technol Assess 2003;7(40).

15. Paisley S, Beard S, Hunn A, Wight J. Clinical effectiveness of oral treatments for spasticity in multiple sclerosis: a systematic review. Mult Scler 2002;8:319–29.

16. Cartlidge NE, Hudgson P, Weightman D. A comparison of baclofen and diazepam in the treatment of spasticity. J Neurol Sci 1974;23:17–24.

17. From A, Heltberg A. A double-blind trial with baclofen (Lioresal) and diazepam in spasticity due to multiple sclerosis. Acta Neurol Scand 1975;51:158–66.

18. Roussan M, Terence C, Fromm G. Baclofen versus diazepam for the treatment of spasticity and long-term follow-up of baclofen therapy. Pharmatherapeutica 1985;5:278–84.

19. Hattab JR. Review of European clinical trials with baclofen. In: Feldman RG, Young RR, Koella WP (eds). Spasticity: Disordered Motor Control. Chicago, IL: Year Book, 1980:71–85.

20. Roy CW, Wakefield IR. Baclofen pseudopsychosis: case report. Paraplegia 1986;24:318–21.

21. Ryan DM, Blumenthal FS. Baclofen-induced dyskinesia. Arch Phys Med Rehabil 1993;74:766–7.

22. Terrence DV, Fromm GH. Complications of baclofen withdrawal. Arch Neurol 1981;38:588–9.

23. Smith CR, La Rocca NG, Giesser BS, Scheinberg LC. High-dose oral baclofen: experience in patients with multiple sclerosis. Neurology 1991;41:1829–31.

24. Coward DM. Tizanidine: neuropharmacology and mechanism of action. Neurology 1994;44(11 Suppl 9):S6–11.

25. Abruzzese G. The medical management of spasticity. Eur J Neurol 2002;9(Suppl 1):30–4.

26. Nance PW, Shears AH, Nance DM. Reflex changes induced by clonidine in spinal cord injured patients. Paraplegia 1989;27:296–301.

27. Meythaler JM, Guin-Refroe S, Johnson A, Brunner RM. Prospective assessment of tizanidine for spasticity due to acquired brain injury. Arch Phys Med Rehabil 2001;82:1155–63.

28. Ward A, Chaffman MO, Sorkin EM. Dantrolene: a review of its pharmokinetic properties and therapeutic use in malignant hyperthermia, the neuroleptic malignant syndrome and an update of its use in muscle spasticity. Drugs 1986;32:130–68.

29. Herman R, Mayer N, Mecomber SA. Clinical pharmaco-physiology of dantrolene sodium. Am J Phys Med 1972;51:296–311.

30. Pinder RM, Brogden RN, Speight TM, Avery GS. Dantrolene sodium: a review of its pharmacological properties and therapeutic effect in spasticity. Drugs 1977;13:3–23.

31. Monster AW. Spasticity and the effect of dantrolene sodium. Arch Phys Medi Rehabil 1974;55:373–83.

32. Schmidt RT, Lee RH, Spehlmann R. Comparison of dantrolene sodium and diazepam in the treatment of spasticity. J Neurol Neurosurg Psychiatry 1976;39:350–6.

33. Weiser R, Terenty T, Hudgson P, Weightman D. Dantrolene sodium in the treatment of spasticity in chronic spinal cord disease. Practitioner 1978;221:123–7.

34. Ketel WB, Kolb ME. Long-term treatment with dantrolene sodium of stroke patients with spasticity limiting the return of function. Curr Med Res Opin 1984;9:161–9.

35. Katrak PH, Cole AMD, Poulos CJ, McCauley JCK. Objective assessment of spasticity, strength, and function with early exhibition of dantrolene sodium after cerebrovascular accident: a randomised double-blind controlled study. Arch Phys Med Rehabil 1992;73:4–9.

36. Haslam RHA, Walcher JR, Lietman PS et al. Dantrolene sodium in children with spasticity. Arch Phys Med Rehabil 1974;55:383–8.

37. Mai J, Pederson E. Mode of action of dantrolene sodium in spasticity. Acta Neurol Scand 1979;59:309–16.

38. Wilson LA, McKechnie AA. Oral diazepam in the treatment of spasticity in paraplegia: a double blind trial and subsequent impressions. Scott Med J 1966;11:46–51.

39. Corbett M, Frankel HL, Michaelis L. A double-blind cross-over trial of valium in the treatment of spasticity. Paraplegia 1972;10:19–22.

40. Cook JB, Nathan PW. On the site of action of diazepam on spasticity in man. J Neurol Sci 1967;5:33–7.

41. Costa E, Guidotti A. Molecular mechanisms in the receptor action of the benzodiazepines. Annu Rev Pharmacol Toxicol 1979;19:531–45.

42. Olsen RW. GABA–benzodiazepine–barbiturate receptor interactions. J Neurochem 1987;37:1–13.

43. March HO. Diazepam in incapacitated cerebral palsied children. JAMA 1965;191:797–800.

44. Engle HA. The effect of diazepam (Valium) in children with cerebral palsy: a double-blind study. Devel Med Child Neurol 1966;8:661–7.

45. Geller A. Common addictions. Clin Symp 1996;48:23–24.

46. Alden KJ, Garcia J. Differential effect of gabapentin on neuronal and muscle calcium currents. J Pharmacol Exp Ther 2001;297:727–35.

47. Czapinski P, Blaszczyk B, Czuczwar SJ. Mechanisms of action of antiepileptic drugs. Curr Top Med Chem 2005;5:3–14.

48. Maneuf YP, Gonzalez MI, Sutton KS et al. Cellular and molecular action of the putative GABA-mimetic, gabapentin. Cell Mol Life Sci 2003;60:742–50.

49. Mueller ME, Gruenthal M, Olson WL, Olson WH. Gabapentin for relief of upper motor neuron symptoms in multiple sclerosis. Arch Phys Med Rehabil 1997;78:521–4.

50. Cutter NC, Scott DD, Johnson JC, Whiteneck G. Gabapentin effect on spasticity in multiple sclerosis: a placebo-controlled, randomised trial. Arch Phys Med Rehabil 2000;81:164–9.

51. Gruenthal M, Mueller M, Olson WL et al. Gabapentin for the treatment of spasticity in patients with spinal cord injury. Spinal Cord 1997;35:686–9.

52. Formica A, Verger K, Sol JM, Morralla C. Gabapentin for spasticity: a randomised, double-blind, placebo-controlled trial. Med Clin (Barc) 2005;124:81–5.

53. Beydoun A, Uthman BM, Sackellares JC. Gabapentin: pharmacokinetics, efficacy, and safety. Clin Neuropharmacol 1995;18:469–81.

54. Baker D, Pryce G, Giavannoni G, Thompson AJ. The therapeutic potential of cannabis. Lancet Neurol 2003;2:291–8.

55. Howlett AC, Barth F, Bonner TI et al. International Union of Pharmacology: XXVII, Classification of Cannabinoid Receptors. Pharmacol Rev 2002;54:161–202.

56. Wilson RI, Nicoll RA. Endocannabinoid signalling in the brain. Science 2002;296:678–82.

57. Wade DT, Robson P, House H et al. A preliminary controlled study to determine whether whole-plant cannabis extracts can improve intractable neurogenic symptoms. Clin Rehabil 2003;17:21–9.

58. Wade DT, Makela P, Robson P et al. Do cannabis-based medicinal extracts have general or specific effects on symptoms in multiple sclerosis? A double-blind, randomised, placebo-controlled study on 160 patients. Mult Scler 2004;10:434–41.

59. Zajicek J, Fox P, Sanders H et al. Cannabinoids for treatment of spasticity and other symptoms related to multiple sclerosis (CAMS study): multicentre randomised placebo-controlled trial. Lancet 2003;362:1517–26.

60. Fox P, Bain PG, Glickman S et al. The effect of cannabis on tremor in patients with multiple sclerosis. Neurology 2004;62:1105–9.

61. Metz L, Page S. Oral cannabinoids for spasticity in multiple sclerosis: will attitude continue to limit use? Lancet 2003;362:1513.

62. Vaney C, Heinzel-Gutenbrunner M, Jobin P et al. Efficacy, safety and tolerability of an orally adminis-tered cannabis extract in the treatment of spasticity in patients with multiple sclerosis: a randomised, double-blind, placebo-controlled, crossover study. Mult Scler 2004;10:417–42.

63. Brady CM, DasGupta R, Dalton C et al. An open-label pilot study of cannabis-based extracts for bladder dysfunction in advanced multiple sclerosis. Mult Scler 2004;10:425–33.

64. Zajicek JP, Sanders HP, Wright DE et al. Cannabinoids in Multiple Sclerosis (CAMS) study: safety and efficacy data for 12 months follow-up. J Neurol Neurosurg Psychiatry 2005;76:1664–9.

65. Kumar RN, Chambers WA, Pertwee RG. Pharmacological action and therapeutic uses of cannabis and cannabinoids. Anaesthesia 2001;56:1059–68.

66. Smith PF. Cannabinoids in the treatment of pain and spasticity in multiple sclerosis. Curr Opin Invest Drugs 2002;3:859–64.

67. Nance PW, Bugaresti J, Shellenberger K et al, and the North American Tizanidine Study Group. Efficacy and safety of tizanidine in the treatment of spasticity in patients with spinal cord injury. Neurology 1994;44(Suppl 9):44–52.

68. Weingarden SI, Belen JG. Clonidine transdermal system for treatment of spasticity in spinal cord injury. Arch Phys Med Rehabil 1992;73:876–7.

69. Hawker K, Frohman E, Racke M. Levetiracetam for phasic spasticity in multiple sclerosis. Arch Neurol 2003;60:1772–4.

70. Grant SM, Heel RC. Vigabatrin – a review of its pharmacodynamic and pharmacokinetic properties and therapeutic potential in epilepsy and disorders of motor control. Drugs 1991;41:889–926.

71. Potter PJ, Hayes KC, Segal JL et al. Randomised double-blind crossover trial of Fampridine-SR (sustained release 4-aminopyridine) in patients with incomplete spinal cord injury. J Neuro Trauma 1998;15:837–49.

72. Davidoff RA. Antispasticity drugs: mechanisms of action. Ann Neurol 1985;17:107–16.

Chapter 6

Focal treatments, including botulinum toxin

Valerie L Stevenson

Often by ensuring that there is an effective physical management plan in place and by avoiding trigger factors, an individual's spasticity can be managed appropriately without pharmacological or surgical input. However, if this is not the case and spasticity is a particularly focal problem, there are specific strategies available other than oral medication: these include botulinum toxin, focal chemical neurolysis or neurotomies. Similarly, some individuals, although they have a generalised picture that is in the most part being effectively managed with oral medication, are still troubled by a focal problem such as a spastic foot drop that is interfering with function. In such individuals, additional focal treatment can be extremely beneficial and may avoid escalation of oral medication with potential side-effects.

Of the focal treatments available, botulinum toxin is the most widely used and the treatment of first choice. Unlike chemical neurolysis or neurotomies, its clinical effects are entirely reversible.

GENERAL ISSUES WITH FOCAL TREATMENTS

Like all interventions to aid spasticity management, focal treatments must be given in the context of a multidisciplinary management plan with clear goals of treatment. Appropriate education for the individual, and if applicable their family or carers, is essential to aid in decision-making and goal formulation and

to maximise the therapeutic effects. Providing written information including details of the agreed goal can facilitate this process (Appendix 5).

Physiotherapy following the intervention is paramount: this may be for ongoing therapy input e.g. aimed at soft tissue lengthening and antagonist muscle strengthening, or could potentially be a one-off session to teach the individual or carers a stretching regime. Regardless of the degree of input, it is essential that arrangements for physiotherapy are in place before treatment is carried out. Likewise, it is important that services including seating and splinting are responsive to changing needs following therapeutic interventions (see Chapter 4).

BOTULINUM TOXIN

Botulinum toxin (BTX) has been used therapeutically since the 1970s, initially for blepharospasm and strabismus but now for many medical conditions, including dystonia, tremor, pain, urogenital dysfunction, cosmetic uses and spasticity.[1]

Mode of action

Botulinum toxin is the most powerful naturally occurring neurotoxin. It is produced by *Clostridium botulinum*, a gram-negative anaerobic bacterium. If ingested, the characteristic clinical picture of botulism will occur, with a descending flaccid motor paralysis and prominent cranial nerve involvement, leading ultimately to respiratory failure and death.

The effect of the toxin is due to inhibition of release of acetylcholine at the neuromuscular junction. Although this blockade is said to be permanent, the clinical effect of injecting botulinum toxin into a muscle is reversible – predominantly due to nerve sprouting and re-innervation leading to functional recovery of the muscle in a few months.[2]

There are seven serotypes of BTX: A–G. Only types A and B are currently licensed for therapeutic use, although investigations into the use of the other serotypes are ongoing. The mechanism of action of BTX is outlined in Figure 6.1. The toxins each comprise of a light and a heavy chain linked together by a disulphide bond. Each serotype binds to a specific site on the presynaptic nerve terminal by its antigen-specific heavy chain. Following internalisation, the disulphide bond is cleaved and the light chain exerts a pathological effect through interrupting membrane fusion and inhibiting calcium-mediated release of acetylcholine. It does this by acting as a zinc-dependent endopeptidase, which cleaves specific proteins within the cytosol, including those of the SNARE (soluble *N*-ethylmaleimide-sensitive factor attachment protein receptors) complex responsible for membrane fusion. Each BTX serotype cleaves one of the SNARE proteins at a specific amino acid site, with a common result of impaired membrane fusion and thereby prevention of release of acetylcholine within the synaptic cleft.[3] Once the BTX has bound to the neurone, the process is irreversible: antitoxin will only be effective against any unbound BTX. In time, there is axonal sprouting and the emergence of new neuromuscular junctions, as well as some recovery of the original junction (perhaps through degradation of the abnormal SNARE protein), accounting for the reversible clinical response (Figure 6.1).

Although the above process begins at the time of injection, the clinical effect of BTX is not apparent immediately and may take up to 10–14 days to have a visible effect. There is some evidence that increasing muscle activity either through voluntary action or by electrical stimulation can potentiate this effect, suggesting that the toxin will 'target' the most overactive fibres.[4,5] If an effect is not seen, it may be that the dose was insufficient or the wrong muscle injected; however, neutralising antibody production against the toxin has also been documented and is probably more common than initially thought. This is of particular concern in so-called 'secondary non-responders' who initially had a good response to BTX injections but then failed to respond. In these individuals, switching to a different preparation of BTX serotype A (BTX-A), or to a different serotype such as BTX-B, may be helpful. To try to limit the development of neutralising antibodies, it is advisable to use the lowest dose that is clinically effective and to avoid injections at intervals of less than 3 months.[6]

Evidence base

Several randomised controlled trials have demonstrated that BTX is effective in reducing tone in stroke, multiple sclerosis (MS), cerebral palsy and head injury; however, few have shown any improvement in active function, although changes in passive function such as ease of hygiene and dressing have been demonstrated. Whether the lack of evidence of functional improvement in some of these studies is truly due to a failure of BTX therapy to impact on function or whether it is related to poor trial design and the lack of function-based outcome measures is difficult to ascertain.[7]

Many of the earlier trials considered patients with spasticity from differing aetiologies, making extrapolation of results to clinical practice difficult. More recently, trials have concentrated on specific patient groups and have focused on potential improvements in function rather than simply the reduction of tone. Unless specified otherwise, all of the trials discussed in this chapter have been performed with BTX-A.

Stroke

Studies of BTX-A in stroke, as in other conditions, are limited in their design, as by definition standardised treatment regimes for therapeutic trials preclude the targeting of optimum muscles personalised for the individual; nonetheless, results are encouraging.[8] Open-label studies in people with upper-limb spasticity secondary to stroke have consistently shown a reduction in tone;[9–11] however, reports of functional improvement in trial participants is limited, with, for example, an increase in ease of personal care reported in one study.[9] Several randomised double-blind placebo-controlled trials have also been completed: again, these have demonstrated an improvement in spasticity scores but only minor effects on function measured by global response scores or a reduction in

Figure 6.1

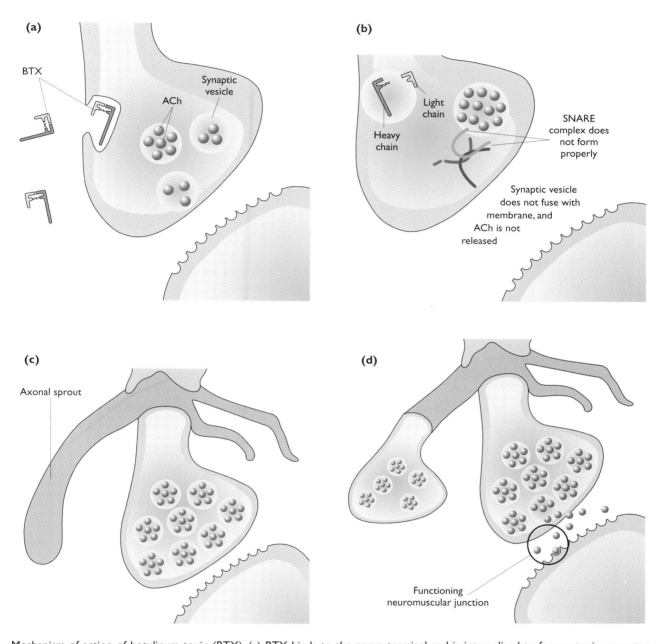

Mechanism of action of botulinum toxin (BTX). (a) BTX binds to the nerve terminal and is internalised to form a toxin–receptor vesicle inside the cell. (b) The light chain of the molecule is then released into the cell cytoplasm and cleaves a SNARE (soluble *N*-ethylmaleimide-sensitive factor attachment protein receptors) protein, preventing the SNARE complex from forming. (c) Axonal sprouting and endplate region growth occurs. (d) Sprouts may then begin to release acetylcholine, forming a new neuromuscular junction. Eventually, the original junction resumes activity, and sprouts regress. Ach, acetylcholine. Reproduced with permission from Allergan

carer burden.[12–17] A notable exception is the study by Brashear et al,[18] which demonstrated a reduction of spasticity in the wrist and fingers of patients following stroke, together with an improvement in their disability assessment scale.

Studies of lower-limb spasticity following stroke have similarly demonstrated a reduction in spasticity scores,[19,20] but also an improvement in a physician rating of gait and a reduction in dependency on walking aids, although there was no change in gait velocity.[20]

The response to BTX-A of post-stroke spasticity in the upper or lower limbs appears to be dose-related, although, not surprisingly, side-effects are more frequent at higher doses.[17,21,22]

Recent studies have also investigated whether combining BTX with electrical stimulation is advantageous. In a short-term study of 24 patients treated with either BTX-A or placebo, with or without 3 days of electrical stimulation, the combined-treatment groups were shown to have greater effects on passive function, such as palm hygiene.[23] Similarly, in a longer-term study of BTX versus BTX in combination with functional electrical stimulation (FES) over a 16-week period, the FES-treated group showed additional benefit, with a significant increase in walking speed.[24]

Little information is as yet available about the long-term efficacy of repeated treatment cycles with BTX. One open-label study assessed 41 individuals with upper-limb spasticity following stroke over three treatment cycles at 12–16-week intervals. No reduction in effect of the BTX-A was seen over this time period and no patients developed neutralising antibodies.[25] Likewise in a larger open-label follow-up study to a double-blind treatment trial in 110 patients,[18] repeated treatments (average of 2.8 per patient) continued to be effective. Only one individual tested positive for neutralising antibodies, and these were present after the first of four treatments with BTX-A, to none of which they responded.[26]

Given the recent interest in other BTX serotypes, Brashear et al[27] have studied the effect of BTX-B on post-stroke upper limb spasticity: no effect was demonstrated on spasticity or function at a dose of 10 000 u.

Multiple sclerosis

There are only two studies assessing the efficacy of BTX-A solely in an MS population, both of which

looked specifically at hip adductor tone.[28,29] Both studies showed a significant reduction in spasticity and an improvement in passive function, particularly perineal hygiene.

Other studies have looked at mixed patient groups: as before, the general effect appears to be a reduction in tone, with some evidence of benefit in passive function (nursing care) but no clear active functional benefit.[30–32]

It is relevant, however, that most patients included in these studies were significantly disabled and therefore it is difficult to extrapolate the findings to ambulant individuals who may be more vulnerable to the adverse effect of increased muscle weakness.[33]

Traumatic brain injury

As with the studies in stroke and MS, BTX has been found to be beneficial in reducing tone in both upper and lower limbs post head injury, with some effect on gait analysis scores.[34,35]

Several studies, although encouraging, are potentially confounded by the fact that casting was employed along with BTX therapy, making it difficult to establish the contribution of the BTX alone to reduction in spasticity.[36–38] However, in one study of 35 patients, there was no significant additional benefit of BTX injections to casting, although further studies were advocated.[38]

Spinal cord injury

Few studies have looked specifically at BTX therapy for managing spasticity in this population; however, it is generally accepted from the studies with mixed cases that BTX can be beneficial in reducing tone and may improve function.[30,34,39,40]

Cerebral palsy

BTX has been trialled in children with cerebral palsy since the early 1990s.[41] Initially, the lower limb was targeted, and as multiple injection sites were necessary, this required a general anaesthetic for the child. As injection regimes were refined, the first randomised controlled trials appeared. In a trial of the hemiplegic upper limb, BTX-A was shown to be effective at reducing muscle tone; subjective scores of beneficial outcome were also positive, but functional outcome measures were equivocal.[42] In the 2004 Cochrane review, only one further randomised controlled trial was considered to be of sufficient quality to consider the efficacy of BTX treatment in the upper limb of children with spastic cerebral palsy.[43] This compared BTX and occupational therapy with occupational therapy alone in 29 children, with a trend for a beneficial effect for the additional use of BTX in a score of quality of movement.[44]

In the lower limb, several studies have looked specifically at the spastic drop foot or equinus deformity. Most trials have shown a beneficial response, with improvement in tone and ambulatory scores.[45–48] Serial casting and splinting has always been the mainstay in the management of the spastic foot drop in cerebral palsy, although it is an inconvenient strategy for both children and their carers or parents. In comparison studies with BTX, both have been shown to be of similar efficacy, but BTX was generally preferred by parents.[49,50] However, in a more recent study, no additional benefit was seen for BTX.[51] Other gait disorders are more complex, and often require an individualised treatment plan with injections at several levels.[52]

It must be remembered that although BTX may be a useful adjunct to physical spasticity management strategies, it is not recommended for long-term use in children. It is generally accepted that younger children show the best response to BTX, and treatment should be considered as part of an overall management plan at an early age. Physical management of these children with stretching regimes and orthotics is, however, ultimately the most important strategy to prevent long-term complications, particularly contractures.[53] Due to bodyweight restrictions in paediatric BTX dosage regimes, focal chemical neurolysis in combination with BTX or other pharmaceutical measures can be a useful treatment strategy to limit the overall dose of BTX administered.

Side-effects

BTX injections are given intramuscularly and therefore may be painful, which can be a limiting factor in the repeated use of BTX, particularly in children, in whom general anaesthesia may be required. Most side-effects are, however, minor and transient: these include soreness, redness or bruising at the injection site.

The major side-effect of BTX is actually its therapeutic effect of weakness, which may cause negative functional consequences, with, for example, reduced grip strength or instability when walking. Due to local diffusion, muscles outside those targeted can be affected – this is of particular concern when injecting neck muscles or facial muscles, where dysphagia, ptosis or diplopia can occur. Thankfully, like the therapeutic effects, these sequelae are temporary.

More widespread effects have also been reported, including generalised weakness, fatigue, anaphylaxis and cardiovascular effects (including changes in blood pressure), although these are rare.[54,55]

Preparations and dosage regime

Currently in the UK and Europe, there are three forms of BTX on the market. Botox (Allergan) and Dysport (Ipsen) are both forms of BTX-A, whereas NeuroBloc (Elan) is the BTX-B serotype. Rather confusingly, dosages for each preparation are not comparable; therefore great care is needed to prevent potentially hazardous mistakes when prescribing, particularly if switching preparations. The potency of all botulinum toxins is measured using the mouse unit. This is a standardised method for assessing toxin strength, with 1 mouse unit (U) being the dose necessary to kill 50% of a group of standardised (18–20 g) female Swiss–Webster mice.[56]

Comparing the two forms of BTX-A, a vial of Botox contains 100 U, while a vial of Dysport has 500 U. However, despite the fact that both preparations are measured in mouse units, Dysport is not actually as potent. This disparity stems from the manufacturing and testing process. In practical terms, studies have suggested that 1 U of Botox is equivalent to about 3–4 U of Dysport.[57] However, in a dose comparison study of patients with blepharospasm or cervical dystonia, ratios of mean dose for Dysport to Botox ranged from as low as 2:1 up to 11:1, suggesting that simple dose conversion factors are not applicable.[58] Similarly, NeuroBloc also has a different dosage schedule, with its potency estimated to be 20–50 times less than that of BTX-A.[59] Thus, for example, dosages for cervical dystonia are of the order of 10 000 U of NeuroBloc compared with 500 U of Dysport and up to 200 U of Botox. Maximum total treatment doses for a 3-month period are of the order of 20 000 U for NeuroBloc,[60] 1000 U for Dysport (Ipsen product information) and 400 U for BOTOX.[56]

Both forms of BTX-A are supplied as freeze-dried powders that require reconstitution with sterile saline. NeuroBloc comes as a liquid ready for injection at a concentration of 5000 U/ml; it can be diluted further with sterile normal saline if necessary.

According to the product information, both Botox and Dysport are indicated for the treatment of the symptomatic relief of blepharospasm, hemifacial spasm and idiopathic cervical dystonia. In addition, Botox is indicated for severe hyperhidrosis of the axillae. With regard to spasticity, both are indicated for dynamic equinus foot deformity due to spasticity in ambulant paediatric cerebral palsy patients, 2 years of age or older. Dysport is also indicated for the management of focal spasticity, including the treatment of arm symptoms associated with focal spasticity (from whatever aetiology) in conjunction with physiotherapy, while Botox is indicated for wrist and hand disability due to upper-limb spasticity associated with stroke in adults. Clearly, both are currently used outside their licensed recommendations in routine clinical practice. NeuroBloc is currently only recommended for use in cervical dystonia.

A guide to commonly used dosage regimes is shown in Table 6.1; however, if there is any concern over possible functional consequences to excessive weakness, these should be reduced.

Cautions

Particular caution should be paid to ensure that BTX is not injected into a blood vessel or used in individuals taking anticoagulants such as warfarin or heparin without careful consideration.

Individuals with other known neuromuscular diseases such as a peripheral neuropathy or motor neurone disease or with neuromuscular junctional disorders (e.g. myasthenia gravis or Lambert–Eaton syndrome) should not be treated with BTX. Likewise, it should not be used in conjunction with other agents that interfere with neuromuscular transmission, such as aminoglycoside antibiotics (e.g. gentamycin) or curare-like compounds.

Table 6.1 Average starting doses for BTX-A therapy

Muscle	Action	Botox (mouse units)	Dysport (mouse units)
Pectoralis	Shoulder adduction	100	300
Biceps	Elbow flexion	100	300–400
Brachioradialis		50	150
Flexor carpi radialis	Wrist flexion	50	150
Flexor carpi ulnaris		40–50	150
Flexor digitorum superficialis	Clenched fist	20	100–250
Flexor digitorum profundus		20	100–150
Psoas	Hip flexion	100	300
Medial hamstrings	Knee flexion	100	300
Lateral hamstrings		100	300
Adductor longus/ brevis/magnus	Adduction of thighs	100–200	300–600
Quadriceps	Knee extension	100	300
Gastrocnemius	Plantarflexion and inversion (equinus foot deformity)	100	300
Soleus		100	300
Tibialis posterior		75	200

None of the BTX preparations are advised in pregnancy or during breast-feeding.

Practical issues with botulinum toxin therapy

Most individuals with spasticity have a long-term neurological disorder or disability. In contrast to the management of cervical dystonia, BTX is rarely used continuously as the mainstay of treatment for spasticity. Instead, it can be viewed as a tool to provide a window of opportunity to establish an effective physical management programme with appropriate exercises, stretches and orthotics. To ensure that this is the case, there must be careful liaison with the whole multidisciplinary team before BTX treatment is given. Through our own experience, we have developed an integrated care pathway (ICP) to help guide this process (Appendix 1).

Once a referral has been received by our service for assessment of an individual's spasticity, we endeavour to obtain as much information as possible before any clinic appointment is arranged. This is sought from the individual, their carers or family if appropriate, district nurses, and any treating therapists either currently or in the past, from community- or secondary-care settings. Once we have gathered this information, we will know more about past or current treatments, therapy input and whether the spasticity is more of a generalised or a focal problem. If spasticity is predominantly a focal concern then BTX therapy may be appropriate, and we will go on to the next stages of preparation. The first of these is to rule out any contraindication to BTX therapy; in our experience, the most frequent problem encountered is concurrent prescribing of warfarin. If this is the case, we will liaise with the individual's GP or anticoagulation clinic to arrange for the warfarin to be adjusted if necessary and have a blood test confirming that the International Normalised Ratio (INR) is no higher than 2.5 a couple of days before the planned appointment.[34]

For all individuals attending the clinic potentially for BTX treatment, we will already have in place a physiotherapy appointment with their local community team or outpatient department for between 7 and 14 days following their spasticity clinic appointment. This ensures that if an individual is suitable for BTX therapy and they wish to go ahead, the treatment can be given at the same time as the assessment, eliminating the need for unnecessary additional appointments.

Once the assessment process has been completed and a decision made to proceed to BTX treatment, a goal is agreed with the individual. This is recorded on both the consent form and on the patient information sheet (Appendix 5), which also includes details of the physiotherapy appointment. Once the procedure has been explained, including potential side-effects, the consent form is signed and the injections are administered.

Following treatment, it is essential that there be an efficient feedback system in place to ensure that everybody involved in the individual's care is aware of the goal of treatment and the ongoing management plan; this may also include specialist seating clinics or orthotics, as well as the treating physiotherapist.

Without careful planning of both the BTX treatment and the follow-up therapy, the effect of any intervention will be minimal and certainly not cost-effective.

Injection of botulinum toxin

The toxin is injected directly into the targeted muscle; the efficacy of injections is related to the proximity of the motor endplate.[61] Higher doses of BTX, higher volumes of injection and multiple injection sites will all promote BTX diffusion, which may increase the effect, but can also increase the potential for side-effects by weakening adjacent muscles.[3] Greater accuracy of injections to the most overactive muscles can be achieved by using electromyographic (EMG) guidance; this can be particularly useful for deep or small muscles.

CHEMICAL NEUROLYSIS

Local injection of ethanol or, more commonly, phenol is an alternative option to botulinum toxin for focal spasticity management. As with any other intervention, this must be done in the context of a goal-orientated management plan and in conjunction with physical measures to optimise the effect. Without an adequate stretching programme or the use of splinting or appropriate orthotics, any benefit realised will be short-lived. Education of the individual, and carers or family if applicable, is extremely important. Procedures to ensure rapid re-assessment of splints, orthotics or seating systems must be in place to optimise the effect from focal neurolysis treatments and to avoid any detrimental effects secondary to a change in posture, position or sensation of a limb.

Chemical neurolysis by phenol or alcohol is irreversible and results in destruction of neural tissue by protein coagulation. Injections may be targeted at peripheral nerves or motor points (intramuscular injections aimed at the parts of muscle most sensitive to electrical stimulation). Following the acute phase, where inflammatory changes are seen within the nerve tissue, there is consequent Wallerian degeneration and fibrous scar tissue is formed. There has been much debate over the exact pathological changes, particularly whether there is a selective fibre effect – although histological animal studies suggest that this is not the case.[62,63]

Electrophysiological studies have attempted to elucidate the factors responsible for the reduction of spasticity following phenol injections: the function of all fibres is probably affected, but the most important effect appears to be on the α motor neurones.[64] Following phenol treatment, partial nerve regeneration and sprouting then occurs, so the clinical effect may 'wear off' after several weeks or months. In animal studies, the effects of re-inervation can be seen as early as 2 weeks following the nerve block.[63] If the clinical effect wanes despite appropriate stretching and splinting regimes, the injections can be repeated.

Before permanent chemical neurolysis procedures are carried out, it is possible, and advisable, to perform a local anaesthetic block (usually with bupivacaine), to demonstrate the efficacy of a permanent neurolysis. This is performed in an identical fashion to the phenol treatment, but the effect only lasts a few hours, allowing the individual with spasticity and the multidisciplinary team to assess the potential impact of a permanent block.

If mixed motor and sensory nerves are targeted, the individual may experience numbness or paraesthesiae following the procedure: occasionally this may be painful, but fortunately such symptoms are usually transient. The local anaesthetic trial is a useful tool to demonstrate any possible sensory impairment in an individual before a definitive procedure is undertaken.

Peripheral phenol nerve blocks have been used in individuals with spasticity from many causes, including head injury, stroke, spinal cord injury, cerebral palsy and MS, in several different anatomical sites. The most commonly applied are tibial (medial popliteal) nerve blocks, particularly in the management of children with developing foot deformities, and obturator nerve blocks in ambulatory patients with scissoring gait or to improve ease of perineal hygiene and aid in seating posture.[65]

Localisation of the injection and side-effects

Most phenol neurolysis procedures are carried out percutaneously using an electrical stimulator for guidance, which improves the accuracy of the injection compared with simply relying on surface anatomy landmarks. Open surgical blocks have been performed in the past, but are not usually necessary.[66,67] Local anaesthetic is first infiltrated into cleansed skin, and the precise site of phenol infiltration is then located using a Teflon-coated needle electrode connected to an electrical stimulator through which the phenol can be administered. As the procedure may be uncomfortable and the individual needs to lie still, children may require a brief general anaesthetic.

The most commonly experienced unwanted effect is lack of efficacy – most usually due to poor localisation of the nerve. However, other effects may be secondary to the injection technique (e.g. the risk of haematoma formation or infection) or to the toxic effects of the phenol. Tissue necrosis has been reported, but is extremely rare. Pain and dysaesthesias due to sensory nerve fibre involvement can also occur, but usually subside with time.

Dosage and concentration

There are no clear guidelines regarding the optimum dose or concentration of neurolytic agents: larger volumes of agent may be necessary to achieve a clinical effect when performing motor point blocks compared with neural blocks.

The concentrations of phenol used in reported studies have usually been between 3% and 7%. In an observational study of 56 nerve blocks in 28 people, 4.5% aqueous phenol was shown to be more effective than 3%.[68] The same group suggest that 4.5% phenol is equivalent to 50% ethanol when used for peripheral nerve blocks.[69]

If function is dependent on some preservation of spasticity or there is a risk of weakening a muscle that may negatively impact on function, it may be necessary to titrate the dose by weekly treatments until the desired effect is achieved.[70]

Common injection sites

Tibial nerve

The most common clinical scenario when considering focal neurolysis treatment is management of the spastic drop foot or equinus deformity. If physical measures are unable to manage the spasticity effectively and there is an impact on function, positioning or the risk of contractures then phenol neurolysis can be an extremely effective procedure, with beneficial effects often lasting several months.

The sciatic nerve divides into the common peroneal and tibial nerves proximal to the popliteal fossa. The tibial nerve motor branches supply the gastrocnemius, soleus, tibialis posterior and flexor digitorum longus muscles, as well as the small muscles of the foot through the medial and lateral plantar nerves. Cutaneous branches include the sural nerve supplying the lateral border of the foot and branches of the plantar nerves to the sole of the foot. There is some debate as to where the most appropriate site is for neurolysis. Some authors have advocated tibial nerve blocks in order to also affect the tibialis posterior and thereby reduce spasticity in the invertors of the foot,[71,72] while others prefer to specifically target the motor branches to the soleus, which may be a more effective strategy than targeting those to the gastrocnemius.[73]

The injections are most easily administered with the patient prone.

Obturator nerve

Many individuals with lower-limb spasticity are troubled by adductor spasms or tone. These can interfere with gait, as well as with personal hygiene and perineal access for catheterisation.

The obturator nerve is formed from the ventral branches of the L2, L3 and L4 roots within the psoas muscle; it then enters the pelvis and passes through the obturator canal into the thigh. Different technical approaches have been described, but efficacy rates are reported to be greatly improved through a combined approach of X-ray fluoroscopy and electrical stimulation.[74] By blocking the obturator nerve at the level of the obturator canal, the motor branches to both the superficial and deep adductor muscles are targeted with greater clinical effect.

Studies have confirmed improvements in gait, as well as improvements in spasm and hygiene scores.[74,75]

Femoral nerve

Spasticity of the quadriceps is often implicated in the inability of hemiplegic individuals to release the knee during walking, resulting in a stiff-legged gait. This can be very disabling, particularly limiting the capacity to manage stairs. However, treating quadriceps overactivity is not straightforward, as there is a risk of reducing hip flexor strength (through an effect on the rectus femoris) or of knee buckling resulting in a detrimental effect on walking. For this reason, investigators have explored selective blocks, either by targeting the branches to the vastus lateralis (with or without additional vastus intermedius blockade)[76] or by selective rectus femoris blocks.[70] The results have been encouraging, although rectus femoris blocks were only found to be useful in those individuals with good hip flexion strength prior to treatment.

Musculocutaneous nerve

The most commonly applied neurolysis procedure to the upper limb is blockade of the musculocutaneous nerve to reduce elbow flexor spasticity. The musculocutaneous nerve is a branch of the lateral cord of the brachial plexus and supplies both the biceps and brachialis muscles as well as the sensory supply to the lateral half of the forearm via the lateral cutaneous nerve of the forearm. Although this can be an effective method of reducing spasticity,[77,78] the use of BTX has generally superseded this approach.

THE SURGICAL MANAGEMENT OF SPASTICITY

Surgical techniques are usually reserved for severe spasticity that cannot be adequately managed with medical and physical measures. Treatment can be targeted at peripheral nerves, much the same as peripheral neurolysis, or at the level of the spinal cord, or via neurostimulation within the brain.[79,80]

Peripheral neurotomies can be performed for any motor peripheral nerves, but most commonly the tibial nerve is targeted to relieve spastic equinus foot deformities.[81–83] Selective dorsal rhizotomies involve sectioning some of the rootlets of each targeted dorsal root to reduce the afferent input while preserving sensory and sphincter function. This has been most extensively applied to children with cerebral palsy, with good efficacy and a sustained improvement not only in spasticity but also in function.[84]

Spinal cord surgery to reduce spasticity has also been advocated, although myelotomies are now rarely performed. Surgery to the dorsal root entry zone – so-called microDREZotomy – is, however, performed in selected centres. This consists of series of small incisions (2–3 mm deep) at the cervical or lumbosacral level guided by electrical stimulation. Selected patients are usually severely disabled due to spasticity and spasms, often with intractable pain; in such individuals, the procedure can bring considerable relief.[80]

Neurostimulation of both the spinal cord and cerebellum has been tried for the relief of severe spasticity. The effect appears to be minimal, and for this reason these strategies have not become part of usual practice.

CONCLUSIONS

Focal therapies for spasticity can be a useful adjunct to physical measures within the context of a multidisciplinary management plan including education of the individual about potential trigger factors for their spasticity and an appropriate stretching and strengthening regime. The use of focal treatments such as BTX or chemical neurolysis can also avoid potential systemic side-effects of escalating oral drug regimes.

Of the focal treatments available, BTX is the most widely used and the treatment of first choice. Surgical measures are an option for severe intractable spasticity, but in practice are rarely necessary.

As with all other interventions, careful planning is essential to ensure that there is a specific goal of treatment that is both achievable and valid to the person with spasticity. Follow-up physiotherapy is essential to optimise the effects of treatment, and must be organised before any interventions are carried out.

REFERENCES

1. Schantz EJ, Johnson EA. Botulinum toxin: the story of its development for the treatment of human disease. Perspect Biol Med 1997;40:317–27.

2. Davis EC, Barnes MP. Botulinum toxin and spasticity. J Neurol Neurosurg Psychiatry 2000;69:143–9.

3. Comella CL, Pullman SL. Botulinum toxins in neurological disease. Muscle Nerve 2004;29:628–44.

4. Eleopra R, Tugnoli V, Caniatti L, De Grandis D. Botulinum toxin treatment in the facial muscles of humans: evidence of an action in untreated near muscles by peripheral local diffusion. Neurology 1996;46:1158–60.

5. Chen R, Karp BI, Goldstein SR et al. Effect of muscle activity immediately after botulinum toxin injection for writer's cramp. Mov Disord 1999;14:307–12.

6. Dressler D. Clinical presentation and management of antibody-induced failure of botulinum toxin therapy. Mov Disord 2004;19(Suppl 8):S92–100.

7. Sheean GL. Botulinum treatment of spasticity: Why is it so difficult to show a functional benefit? Curr Opin Neurol 2001;14:771–6.

8. Van Kuijk AA, Geurts ACH, Bevaart BJW, van Limbeek. Treatment of upper extremity spasticity in stroke patients by focal neuronal or neuromuscular blockade: a systematic review of the literature. J Rehabil Med 2002;34:51–61.

9. Hesse S, Friedrich H, Domasch C, Mauritz KH. Botulinum toxin therapy for upper limb spasticity: preliminary results. J Rehabil Sci 1992;5:98–101.

10. Bhakta BB, Cozens JA, Bamford JM, Chamberlain MA. Use of botulinum toxin in stroke patients with severe upper limb spasticity. J Neurol Neurosurg Psychiatry 1996;61:30–5.

11. Sampaio C, Ferreira JJ, Pinto AA et al. Botulinum toxin type A for the treatment of arm and hand spasticity in stroke patients. Clin Rehabil 1997;11:3–7.

12. Simpson DM, Alexander DN, O'Brien CF et al. Botulinum toxin type A in the treatment of upper extremity spasticity: a randomised, double-blind, placebo-controlled trial. Neurology 1996;46:1306–10.

13. Bakheit AM, Thilmann AF, Ward AB et al. A randomised, double-blind, placebo-controlled, dose-ranging study to compare the efficacy and safety of three doses of botulinum toxin type A (Dysport) with placebo in upper limb spasticity after stroke. Stroke 2000;31:2402–6.

14. Bhakta BB, Cozens JA, Chamberlain MA, Bamford JM. Impact of botulinum toxin type A on disability and carer burden due to arm spasticity after stroke: a randomised double blind placebo controlled trial. J Neurol Neurosurg Psychiatry 2000;69:217–21.

15. Smith SJ, Ellis E, White S, Moore AP. A double-blind placebo-controlled study of botulinum toxin in upper limb spasticity after stroke or head injury. Clin Rehabil 2000;14:5–13.

16. Bakheit AM, Pittock S, Moore AP et al. A randomised, double-blind, placebo-controlled study of

the efficacy and safety of botulinum toxin type A in upper limb spasticity in patients with stroke. Eur J Neurol 2001;8:559–65.

17. Childers MK, Brashear A, Jozefczyk P et al. Dose-dependent response to intramuscular botulinum toxin type A for upper-limb spasticity in patients after a stroke. Arch Phys Med Rehabil 2004;85:1063–9.

18. Brashear A, Gordon MF, Elovic E et al. Intramuscular injection of botulinum toxin for the treatment of wrist and finger spasticity after a stroke. N Engl J Med 2002;347:395–400.

19. Hesse S, Lucke D, Malezic M et al. Botulinum toxin treatment for lower limb extensor spasticity in chronic hemiparetic patients. J Neurol Neurosurg Psychiatry 1994;57:1321–4.

20. Burbaud P, Wiart L, Dubos JL et al. A randomised, double blind, placebo controlled trial of botulinum toxin in the treatment of spastic foot in hemiparetic patients. J Neurol Neurosurg Psychiatry 1996;61:265–9.

21. Pittock SJ, Moore AP, Hardiman O et al. A double-blind randomised placebo-controlled evaluation of three doses of botulinum toxin type A (Dysport) in the treatment of spastic equinovarus deformity after stroke. Cerebrovasc Dis 2003;15:289–300.

22. Mancini F, Sandrini G, Moglia A et al. A randomised, double-blind, dose-ranging study to evaluate efficacy and safety of three doses of botulinum toxin type A (Botox) for the treatment of spastic foot. Neurol Sci 2005;26:26–31.

23. Hesse S, Reiter F, Konrad M, Jahnke MT. Botulinum toxin type A and short-term electrical stimulation in the treatment of upper limb flexor spasticity after stroke: a randomised, double-blind, placebo-controlled trial. Clin Rehabil 1998;12:381–8.

24. Johnson CA, Burridge JH, Strike PW et al. The effect of combined use of botulinum toxin type A and functional electric stimulation in the treatment of spastic drop foot after stroke: a preliminary investigation. Arch Phys Med Rehabil 2004;85:902–9.

25. Bakheit AM, Fedorova NV, Skoromets AA et al. The beneficial antispasticity effect of botulinum toxin type A is maintained after repeated treatment cycles. J Neurol Neurosurg Psychiatry 2004;75:1558–61.

26. Gordon MF, Brashear A, Elovic E et al. Repeated dosing of botulinum toxin type A for upper limb spasticity following stroke. Neurology 2004;63:1971–3.

27. Brashear A, McAfee AL, Kuhn ER, Fyffe J. Botulinum toxin type B in upper-limb poststroke spasticity: a double-blind, placebo-controlled trial. Arch Phys Med Rehabil 2004;85:705–9.

28. Snow BJ, Tsui JKC, Bhatt MH et al. Treatment of spasticity with botulinum toxin: a double blind study. Ann Neurol 1990;28:512–15.

29. Hyman N, Barnes M, Bhakta B et al. Botulinum toxin (Dysport) treatment of hip adductor spasticity in multiple sclerosis: a prospective, randomised, double blind, placebo controlled, dose ranging study. J Neurol Neurosurg Psychiatry 2000;68:707–12.

30. Dunne JW, Heye N, Dunne SL. Treatment of chronic limb spasticity with botulinum toxin A. J Neurol Neurosurg Psychiatry 1995;58:232–5.

31. Grazko MA, Polo KB, Jabbari B. Botulinum toxin A for spasticity, muscle spasms, and rigidity. Neurology 1995;45:712–17.

32. Cava TJ. Botulinum toxin management of spasticity in upper motor neuron lesions. Eur J Neurol 1995;2:57–60.

33. Beard S, Hunn A, Wight J. Treatments for spasticity and pain in multiple sclerosis: a systematic review. Health Technol Assess 2003;7(40).

34. Richardson D, Sheean G, Werring D et al. Evaluating the role of botulinum toxin in the management of focal hypertonia in adults. J Neurol Neurosurg Psychiatry 2000;69:499–506.

35. Fock J, Galea MP, Stillman BC et al. Functional outcome following botulinum toxin A injection to reduce spastic equinus in adults with traumatic brain injury. Brain Inj 2004;18:57–63.

36. Yablon SA, Agana BT, Ivanhoe CB, Boake C. Botulinum toxin in severe upper extremity spasticity among patients with traumatic brain injury: an open labelled trial. Neurology 1996;47:939–44.

37. Pavesi G, Brianti R, Medici D et al. Botulinum toxin type A in the treatment of upper limb spasticity among patients with traumatic brain injury. J Neurol Neurosurg Psychiatry 1998;64:419–20.

38. Verplancke D, Snape S, Salisbury CF et al. A randomised controlled trial of botulinum toxin on lower limb spasticity following acute acquired severe brain injury. Clin Rehabil 2005;19:117–25.

39. Fried GW, Fried KM. Spinal cord injury and use of botulinum toxin in reducing spasticity. Phys Med Rehabil Clin N Am 2003;14:901–10.

40. Richardson D, Edwards S, Sheean GL et al. The effect of botulinum toxin on hand function after incomplete spinal cord injury at C5/6: a case report. Clin Rehabil 1997;11:288–92.

41. Cosgrove AP, Corry IS, Graham HK. Botulinum toxin in the management of the lower limb in cerebral palsy. Dev Med Child Neurol 1994;36:386–96.

42. Corry IS, Cosgrove AP, Walsh EG et al. Botulinum toxin A in the hemiplegic upper limb: a double-blind trial. Dev Med Child Neurol 1997;39:185–93.

43. Wasiak J, Hoare B, Wallen M. Botulinum toxin A as an adjunct to treatment in the management of the upper limb in children with spastic cerebral palsy. Cochrane Database Syst Rev 2004;(3):CD003469.

44. Fehlings D, Rang M, Glazier J, Steele C. An evaluation of botulinum-A toxin injections to improve upper extremity function in children with hemiplegic cerebral palsy. J Pediatr 2000;137:331–7.

45. Koman LA, Mooney JF 3rd, Smith BP et al. Botulinum toxin type A neuromuscular blockade in the treatment of lower extremity spasticity in cerebral palsy: a randomised, double-blind, placebo-controlled trial. BOTOX Study Group. J Pediatr Orthop 2000;20:108–15.

46. Koman LA, Brashear A, Rosenfeld S et al. Botulinum toxin type A neuromuscular blockade in the treatment of equinus foot deformity in cerebral palsy: a multicenter, open-label clinical trial. Pediatrics 2001;108:1062–71.

47. Baker R, Jasinski M, Maciag-Tymecka I et al. Botulinum toxin treatment of spasticity in diplegic cerebral palsy: a randomised, double-blind, placebo-controlled, dose-ranging study. Dev Med Child Neurol 2002;44:666–75.

48. Satila H, Iisalo T, Pietikainen T et al. Botulinum toxin treatment of spastic equinus in cerebral palsy: a randomised trial comparing two injection sites. Am J Phys Med Rehabil 2005;84:355–65.

49. Corry IS, Cosgrove AP, Duffy CM et al. Botulinum toxin A compared with stretching casts in the treatment of spastic equinus: a randomised prospective trial. J Pediatr Orthop 1998;18:304–11.

50. Flett PJ, Stern LM, Waddy H et al. Botulinum toxin A versus fixed cast stretching for dynamic calf tightness in cerebral palsy. J Paediatr Child Health 1999;35:71–7.

51. Kay RM, Rethlefsen SA, Fern-Buneo A et al. Botulinum toxin as an adjunct to serial casting treatment in children with cerebral palsy. J Bone Joint Surg Am 2004;86–A:2377–84.

52. Pirpiris M, Graham HK. Management of spasticity in children. In: Barnes MP, Johnson GR (eds). Upper Motor Neurone Syndrome and Spasticity: Clinical Management and Neurophysiology. Cambridge: Cambridge University Press, 2001: 266–305.

53. Koman LA, Smith BP, Shilt JS. Cerebral palsy. Lancet 2004;363:1619–31.

54. Bakheit AMO, Ward CD, McLellan DL. Generalised botulism-like syndrome after intramuscular injections of botulinum toxin type A: a report of two cases. J Neurol Neurosurg Psychiatry 1997;62:198.

55. Bhatia KP, Munchau A, Thompson PD et al. Generalised muscular weakness after botulinum toxin injections for dystonia: a report of three cases. J Neurol Neurosurg Psychiatry 1999;67:90–3.

56. Brin MF. Botulinum toxin: chemistry, pharmacology, toxicity and immunology. Muscle Nerve 1997;Suppl 6:S146–68.

57. Wohlfarth K, Kampe K, Bigalke H. Pharmacokinetic properties of different formulations of botulinum neurotoxin type A. Mov Disord 2004;19(Suppl 8):S65–7.

58. Marchetti A, Magar R, Findley L et al. Retrospective evaluation of the dose of dysport and BOTOX in the management of cervical dystonia and blepharospasm: The REAL DOSE study. Mov Disord 2005;20:937–44.

59. Sloop RR, Cole BA, Escutin RO. Human response to botulinum toxin injection: type B compared with type A. Neurology 1997;49:189–94.

60. Berman B, Seeberger L, Kumar R. Long-term safety, efficacy, dosing, and development of resistance with botulinum toxin type B in cervical dystonia. Mov Disord 2005;20:233–7.

61. Shaari CM, Sanders I. Quantifying how location and dose of botulinum toxin injections affect muscle paralysis. Muscle Nerve 1993;16:964–9.

62. Burkel WE, McPhee M. Effect of phenol injection into peripheral nerve of rat: electron microscope studies. Arch Phys Med Rehabil 1970;49:333–47.

63. Bodine-Fowler SC, Allsing S, Botte MJ. Time course of muscle atrophy and recovery following a phenol-induced nerve block. Muscle Nerve 1996;19:497–504.

64. On AY, Kirazli Y, Kismali B, Aksit R. Mechanisms of action of phenol block and botulinus toxin type A in relieving spasticity: electrophysiologic investigation and follow up. Am J Phys Med Rehabil 1999;78:344–9.

65. Barnes MP. Local treatment of spasticity. Baillieres Clin Neurol 1993;2:55–71.

66. Garland DE, Lucie RS, Waters RL. Current uses of open phenol nerve block for adult acquired spasticity. Clin Orthop Rel Res 1982;165:217–22.

67. Moore TJ, Anderson RB. The use of open phenol blocks to the motor branches of the tibial nerve in adult acquired spasticity. Foot Ankle 1991;11:219–21.

68. Bakheit AMO, Badwan DAH, McLellan DL. The effectiveness of chemical neurolysis in the treatment of lower limb muscle spasticity. Clin Rehabil 1996;10:40–3.

69. Bakheit AMO, McLellan DL, Burnett ME. Symptomatic and functional improvement in foot dystonia with medial popliteal nerve block. Clin Rehabil 1996;10:347–9.

70. Sung DH, Bang HJ. Motor branch block of the rectus femoris: Its effectiveness in stiff-legged gait in spastic paresis. Arch Phys Med Rehabil 2000;81:910–15.

71. Petrillo CR, Knoploch S. Phenol block of the tibial nerve for spasticity: a long-term follow-up study. Int Disabil Stud 1988;10:97–100.

72. Kirazli Y, On AY, Kismali B, Aksit R. Comparison of phenol block and botulinus toxin type A in the treatment of spastic foot after stroke: a randomised, double-blind trial. Am J Phys Med Rehabil 1998;77:510–15.

73. Buffenoir K, Decq P, Lefaucheur JP. Interest of peripheral anesthetic blocks as a diagnosis and prognosis tool in patients with spastic equinus foot: a clinical and electrophysiological study of the effects of block of nerve branches to the triceps surae muscle. Clin Neurophysiol 2005;116:1596–600.

74. Viel EJ, Perennou D, Ripart J et al. Neurolytic blockade of the obturator nerve for intractable spasticity of adductor thigh muscles. Eur J Pain 2002;6:97–104.

75. Ofluoglu D, Esquenazi A, Hirai B. Temporospatial parameters of gait after obturator neurolysis in patients with spasticity. Am J Phys Med Rehabil 2003;82:832–6.

76. Albert TA, Yelnik A, Bonan I et al. Effectiveness of femoral nerve selective block in patients with spasticity: preliminary results. Arch Phys Med Rehabil 2002;83:692–6.

77. Keenan MA, Tomas ES, Stone L, Gersten LM. Percutaneous phenol block of the musculocutaneous nerve to control elbow flexor spasticity. J Hand Surg 1990;15:340–6.

78. Kong KH, Chua KSG. Neurolysis of the musculocutaneous nerve with alcohol to treat poststroke elbow flexor spasticity. Arch Phys Med Rehabil 1999;80:1234–6.

79. Lazorthes Y, Sol JC, Sallerin B, Verdie JC. The surgical management of spasticity. Eur J Neurol 2002;9 (Suppl 1):35–41.

80. Mertens P, Sindou M. Surgical management of spasticity. In: Barnes MP, Johnson GR (eds). Upper Motor Neurone Syndrome and Spasticity: Clinical Management and Neurophysiology. Cambridge: Cambridge University Press, 2001: 239–65.

81. Sindou M, Keravel Y. Microsurgical procedures in the peripheral nerves and the dorsal root entry zone for the treatment of spasticity. Scand J Rehabil Med 1988;Suppl 17:139–43.

82. Abdennebi B, Bougatene B. Selective neurotomies for relief of spasticity focalised to the foot and to the knee flexors. Results in a series of 58 patients. Acta Neurochir (Wien) 1996;138:917–20.

83. Decq P, Filipetti P, Cubillos A et al. Soleus neurotomy for treatment of the spastic equinus foot. Groupe d'Evaluation et de Traitement de la Spasticité et de la Dystonie. Neurosurgery 2000;47:1154–61.

84. Mittal S, Farmer JP, Al-Atassi B et al. Long-term functional outcome after selective posterior rhizotomy. J Neurosurg 2002;97:315–25.

Chapter 7

Intrathecal therapies, including baclofen and phenol

Louise Jarrett

Sometimes, despite optimum multidisciplinary input with close attention to minimising trigger or aggravating factors, spasticity cannot be managed appropriately with a combination of physical measures and oral medication alone. As outlined in Chapter 6, focal therapies such as botulinum toxin or peripheral nerve blocks may be useful; however, if the problem is more widespread (such as with bilateral lower limb spasticity) then intrathecal baclofen (ITB) or phenol (IP) are further options to consider.

INTRATHECAL BACLOFEN THERAPY

ITB was first used in 1985 for spinal cord injury[1] and has since been shown to be an effective treatment in the management of severe spasticity of either cerebral[2,3] or spinal origin[4,5] and for specific conditions such as brain injury,[6] multiple sclerosis (MS)[7] and hemiplegia.[8,9] In long-term follow-up studies, the benefit has proved to be sustainable over time,[10–12] with many individuals continuing to benefit following a pump replacement once the battery life of the original pump has been depleted. More recently, it has been used to improve specific functions, such as the speech of a person with cerebral palsy.[13] There has also been interest in the use of ITB in the acute setting of managing severe head injury with associated spasticity and dysautonomias, or so-called 'storming'. Small case series have suggested a benefit for ITB in this setting with positive effects on both spasticity and in the stabilisation of autonomic dysfunction.[6,14]

Mode of action

Baclofen acts by binding to γ-aminobutyric acid (GABA) receptors. It has a presynaptic inhibitory effect on the release of excitatory neurotransmitters[15] and postsynaptically it decreases the firing of motor neurones.[16] This results in inhibition of both mono- and polysynaptic spinal reflexes,[17] with associated reductions in spasticity, spasm, clonus and pain. The purpose of administering doses of baclofen intrathecally is to deliver it directly to the GABA receptors; this accentuates its anti-spasticity effect while minimising the troublesome systemic side-effects sometimes associated with oral intake.

Mode of delivery

Baclofen can be administered intrathecally in the short term via a lumbar puncture or an external lumbar catheter, or for longer-term use via a subcutaneously implanted pump. Different types of pump are available. Some are battery-dependent electronic models that can be programmed by a computer with telemetry, thus enabling the dose to be varied over a 24-hour period. Other pumps use a gas-compression reservoir to provide an inexhaustible energy source, thus delivering a constant dose over the 24-hour period. The advantage of electronic pumps is in the flexibility of the dosage regime, which can be particularly useful when dealing with progressive diseases where spasticity may vary over time. However, constant-flow pumps can be useful where the spasticity is felt to be

Figure 7.1

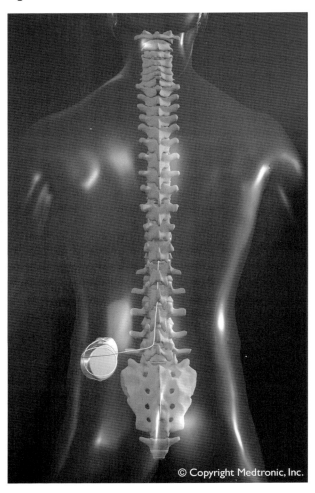

© Copyright Medtronic, Inc.

Position of intrathecal baclofen pump and catheter. Reproduced with permission from Medtronic

Figure 7.2

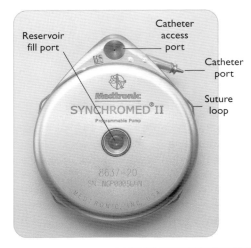

Dimensions of SynchroMed II infusion pump		
	20 ml reservoir	*40 ml reservoir*
Depth	19.5 mm	26 mm
Diameter	87.5 mm	87.5 mm
Weight (empty/full)	165/185 g	175/215 g

Medtronic SynchroMed II infusion system: the pump. Reproduced with permission from Medtronic

static and to require infrequent changes in the doses delivered, with the added benefit of not being battery-dependent.

Despite these differences, the systems have similar components: each pump has a reservoir where the drug is stored and a mechanism to deliver the drug over time; a catheter links the pump to the intrathecal space. The pump is implanted into a subcutaneous abdominal pocket and the catheter into the intrathecal space with the tip situated at L2/L3 or higher, thus allowing the drug to be delivered directly toward the GABA receptors of the spinal cord (Figure 7.1).

Figures 7.2 and 7.3 show parts of the Medtronic SynchroMed infusion system. This system is externally programmed using a handheld computer and telemetry (Figure 7.3), allowing different dose regimes to be delivered. A 24-hour dose can have up

to 10 steps, each prescribing the dose, rate and duration, allowing the delivery of complex regimes. This enables the dose of baclofen delivered to vary throughout the day, reflecting an individual's need throughout the 24-hour period. For example, in an ambulant individual, the daytime dose may be less than overnight, where higher doses are needed to eliminate painful spasms but not at the risk of jeopardising walking. Alternatively, bolus doses can be given prior to a task to ease its completion: for instance, giving a bolus in advance may ease the effort for a person to wash and dress. In this way, regimes can be highly personalised and can be adapted over time if circumstances change.

Current models of these electronic pumps have a battery that depletes after 5–7 years, necessitating an entire pump replacement (if patent, the catheter remains in place). Electronic pumps also tend to have an alarm system that will alert if the reservoir volume is low, the battery is depleted or the pump malfunctions. In addition, it is also possible (in carefully selected individuals) to programme the pump to allow the person themselves to administer a

Figure 7.3

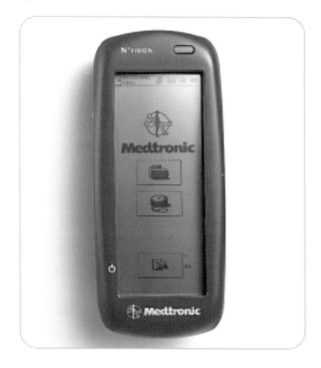

Medtronic SynchroMed II infusion system: the programmer. Reproduced with permission from Medtronic

predefined number of 'rescue' bolus doses by means of a 'patient therapy manager', which acts very similarly to a telemetry patient-controlled analgesia device. The physician determines the size of the bolus and the number of doses allowed within a defined time period.

Provision of a safe ITB service

The use of ITB is not without risk of complications. Therefore setting up a service requires a robust clinical governance framework, where elements of risk are clearly identified and structures are in place to minimise problems while maximising the benefit of ITB therapy. A coordinated approach by an experienced team including a neurologist, neurosurgeon, physiotherapists, nurses, occupational therapists and/or rehabilitation professionals is advisable,[7,18] with appropriate involvement and education of the individual with spasticity at every stage.

The assessment and management processes to allow safe administration of ITB treatment require detailed protocols and guidelines to be developed and regularly reviewed. The ITB service at the National Hospital for Neurology and Neurosurgery (NHNN), London was established over 10 years ago; this chapter reflects the current content of the multidisciplinary protocol, together with guidelines and patient information that have been established and refined over time. These include a patient information leaflet (Appendix 6), the medical procedure for the ITB trial injection (Appendix 7), ITB nursing care plans (Appendix 8), an example of specific competencies for a specialist nurse (Appendix 9), physiotherapy guidelines (Appendix 10), an outline of the surgical procedure (Appendix 11) and details of the refill process (Appendix 12). Although these guidelines have been designed specifically for the services at NHNN, they could easily be adapted to other centres.

Selection process

Selection of people for ITB necessitates a detailed assessment (Chapter 2), during which the optimisation of trigger factors and the effect of management techniques, including physical measures, oral medication and botulinum toxin, are assessed. If it is found that they are no longer effective in managing the spasticity or are thought not to be indicated then ITB can be considered as an option. In acute conditions such as autonomic dysfunction following severe head injury, ITB may be used early, before other treatment options are tried, as an effective mechanism to prevent further brain injury secondary to so-called autonomic storming.[6,14]

When considering ITB as part of a long-term spasticity management plan, criteria can be used to assist in the selection of appropriate candidates for a trial of ITB therapy (Table 7.1). The criteria are best

Table 7.1 Selection criteria for an intrathecal baclofen (ITB) trial

- Severe lower-limb spasticity that impacts on the person's daily life (e.g. Ashworth[45] grade 2 or above and/or Penn[4] scale 2 or above)

- Physical adjuncts, therapy, nursing, the use of oral medication and/or botulinum toxin no longer adequately manage the person's spasticity

- The individual or their carer participate in discussions about ITB, agree to a trial and demonstrate an awareness of the potential long-term commitment involved with ITB therapy

used as a guide alongside detailed assessments, as it is often difficult to accurately predict the effect of ITB prior to doing a trial, even with the benefit of comprehensive assessments and measures in a person who fits the criteria.

Education of the person

Before undertaking ITB therapy, the individual needs to understand what the process involves. This requires detailed explanations of the different stages: the trial, the implant, pump replacement and ongoing follow-up. It is important that the quantity of information and timing of its delivery be paced to the individual's ability to assimilate it (Chapter 3). Different aspects may require repetition and further explanation, perhaps with a relative or carer present. Verbal explanations can be supplemented with written information or with the use of aids such as an imitation pump, and time must be provided for the individual to ask questions. A written information sheet containing appropriate contact details for a member of the team to clarify any issues is essential (Appendix 6).

Individual commitment

Successful ITB therapy is dependent on the individual being fully involved in the assessment and decision-making process. This ensures that the assessment process and identification of an appropriate treatment goal reflect the person's perspective on how the changes in their spasticity and spasms may affect their functioning at home and their overall quality of life. Some individuals also choose to include a significant other to support them in the assessment and decision-making process.

Committing to long-term ITB therapy is not a trivial decision for a person to make, as it involves surgery, adjustment to living with an implant that requires frequent follow-up, and the need to take responsibility for acting promptly if symptoms persist or if side-effects occur. For these reasons, education and involvement of the individual in a rigorous assessment process and intrathecal trial to assist in decision-making is paramount.

The ITB trial

The ITB trial is an integral part of the assessment and decision-making process for potential long-term ITB therapy. This process is illustrated as an algorithm in Figure 7.4.

The trial consists of administering a bolus dose of ITB via lumbar puncture; a detailed medical protocol for the trial injection is detailed in Appendix 7. At least two trials are completed, each on a separate day. The initial dose given is 25 µg, with increments being no more than 25 µg at a time. Even if the person has a response at 25 µg, the trial is usually repeated with 50 µg to confirm a response and help gauge the potential for goal achievement. In some cases, the higher dose produces the same outcome as the lower dose, illustrating the maximal effect of the treatment for that person. This can be useful for the individual to experience, as it can guide them to decide whether the impact is significant enough to proceed to implant. On rare occasions, if excessive weakness underlying the spasticity is exposed with 25 µg, the second dose is halved to 12.5 µg. This occurs predominantly when the aim is to preserve the quality of the individual's walking and their ability to do so whilst minimising some of the negative effects of their spasticity and spasms.

The trial injection permits a relatively large amount of baclofen to enter the intrathecal space rapidly: there is therefore a risk of overdose or other side-effects that necessitates careful monitoring of the individual[19] (Table 7.2). Sensitivity to ITB varies markedly between individuals: signs of severe overdose have been reported after a single test dose of only 25 µg.[20] The peak clinical effect of the drug is usually 4 hours after injection; this period from injection to peak effect is a particularly critical time for the person, who requires vigilant observation and monitoring by nursing staff. It is recommended that the doses be administered with resuscitation equipment readily available and with frequent monitoring of vital signs, oxygen saturation levels and neurological status for at least 6 hours after the injection. Skilled nursing care for the trial is therefore extremely important, and for this reason specific care plans (Appendix 8) and nurse specialist competencies (Appendix 9) have been developed to ensure that the individual is managed appropriately to minimise risk.

To ensure that members of the team are available to manage any side-effects, and to reassess and remeasure the person as the drug peaks after 4 hours, the trial injection is best given before midday. A result is deemed positive if the person experiences a beneficial effect for 6–8 hours post peak time.

Figure 7.4

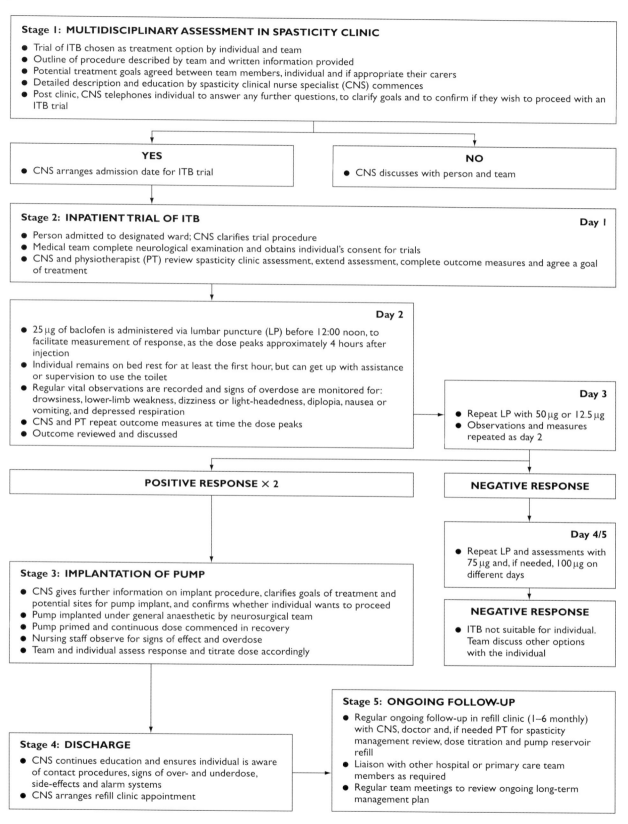

Stage 1: MULTIDISCIPLINARY ASSESSMENT IN SPASTICITY CLINIC
- Trial of ITB chosen as treatment option by individual and team
- Outline of procedure described by team and written information provided
- Potential treatment goals agreed between team members, individual and if appropriate their carers
- Detailed description and education by spasticity clinical nurse specialist (CNS) commences
- Post clinic, CNS telephones individual to answer any further questions, to clarify goals and to confirm if they wish to proceed with an ITB trial

YES
- CNS arranges admission date for ITB trial

NO
- CNS discusses with person and team

Stage 2: INPATIENT TRIAL OF ITB   **Day 1**
- Person admitted to designated ward; CNS clarifies trial procedure
- Medical team complete neurological examination and obtains individual's consent for trials
- CNS and physiotherapist (PT) review spasticity clinic assessment, extend assessment, complete outcome measures and agree a goal of treatment

Day 2
- 25 μg of baclofen is administered via lumbar puncture (LP) before 12:00 noon, to facilitate measurement of response, as the dose peaks approximately 4 hours after injection
- Individual remains on bed rest for at least the first hour, but can get up with assistance or supervision to use the toilet
- Regular vital observations are recorded and signs of overdose are monitored for: drowsiness, lower-limb weakness, dizziness or light-headedness, diplopia, nausea or vomiting, and depressed respiration
- CNS and PT repeat outcome measures at time the dose peaks
- Outcome reviewed and discussed

Day 3
- Repeat LP with 50 μg or 12.5 μg
- Observations and measures repeated as day 2

POSITIVE RESPONSE × 2

NEGATIVE RESPONSE

Day 4/5
- Repeat LP and assessments with 75 μg and, if needed, 100 μg on different days

Stage 3: IMPLANTATION OF PUMP
- CNS gives further information on implant procedure, clarifies goals of treatment and potential sites for pump implant, and confirms whether individual wants to proceed
- Pump implanted under general anaesthetic by neurosurgical team
- Pump primed and continuous dose commenced in recovery
- Nursing staff observe for signs of effect and overdose
- Team and individual assess response and titrate dose accordingly

NEGATIVE RESPONSE
- ITB not suitable for individual. Team discuss other options with the individual

Stage 5: ONGOING FOLLOW-UP
- Regular ongoing follow-up in refill clinic (1–6 monthly) with CNS, doctor and, if needed PT for spasticity management review, dose titration and pump reservoir refill
- Liaison with other hospital or primary care team members as required
- Regular team meetings to review ongoing long-term management plan

Stage 4: DISCHARGE
- CNS continues education and ensures individual is aware of contact procedures, signs of over- and underdose, side-effects and alarm systems
- CNS arranges refill clinic appointment

NHNN algorithm for intrathecal baclofen (ITB) therapy

Table 7.2 Potential side-effects of intrathecal baclofen therapy

Signs of acute overdose	Other side-effects
Drowsiness	Muscle hypotonia
Weakness in lower limbs	Headache
Dizziness/light-headedness	Confusion, hallucinations, mood changes
Diplopia	
Depressed respiration	Seizures
Nausea/vomiting	Hypotension
	Dysphagia, dysarthria
	Nystagmus
	Urinary incontinence or retention
	Ileus, constipation or diarrhoea
	Sexual dysfunction
	Paraesthesia
	Bradycardia
	Allergic reactions
	Peripheral oedema
	Deep-vein thrombosis

Procedure following trial

The team discuss outcomes from both trials collectively with the individual, and their family or carers if appropriate, and decide whether there is a clear positive or negative effect, or whether further trial doses are required to clarify the potential usefulness of ITB therapy. Further doses may be given of 75 µg or 100 µg; if the person does not respond to these doses, they are unlikely to be suitable for ITB therapy due to the risk of inducing side-effects. However, if the trials are successful, the person meets the pump implant selection criteria (Table 7.3) and all concerned agree to go ahead then a pump implant is arranged. Occasionally, individuals are discharged home following the trial and readmitted for pump insertion at a later date, depending on their wishes and the availability of the surgeon. Some individuals prefer to return home equipped with the knowledge from the trial to make a final assessment on how ITB could impact on their lifestyle at home before committing to the pump implant.

Table 7.3 Criteria for intrathecal baclofen (ITB) pump implant

- Severe lower-limb spasticity that impacts on the person's daily life (e.g. Ashworth[45] grade 2 or above and/or Penn[4] scale 2 or above)
- Oral medication, physical adjuncts, therapy and nursing no longer adequately manage the person's spasticity
- The individual responds positively to two ITB trials
- The individual or carer agree with the treatment goals, and are aware of their role in managing and being responsible for the pump
- If a person has a history of drug abuse or self-harm, the future potential risk needs to be considered as minimal by appropriate professionals

It is important to consider whether there are any other medical issues that may impact on the safety of an implantable pump. One such example is that of a history of drug abuse or self-harm: it is of course possible that a person could access the baclofen reservoir relatively easily if they were so inclined, and baclofen or other substances could cause adverse events including respiratory arrest, if injected inappropriately. Similarly, if self-harm is an issue, infected skin lesions or wound contamination can cause potential complications, including infection of the pump system. If there is cause for concern, a psychiatric opinion related to the current and future risk may be pertinent.

If indicated, the issue of potential problems with pregnancy (in particular carrying a foetus to term with a pump in situ) should be discussed. Although not a frequent occurrence, there is one case in the literature where a successful pregnancy occurred with an implanted pump and ongoing ITB therapy seemingly having no adverse effects on the development of the baby.[21] Similarly, with a pregnant woman who developed tetanus, ITB boluses were successfully infused over a 21-day period with no adverse effects on the development of the baby.[22]

Pump implantation

The surgical technique used may vary, depending on the preference of the surgeon: certain aspects of the surgical technique used at the NHNN have been modified over time to make the procedure more effective (Appendix 11).

The most important issue at implant for the follow-up team is that the length of catheter implanted be accurately recorded. This is not only required to calculate the initial priming bolus dose, but is also necessary for future bridging bolus doses, if the concentration of the baclofen inserted into the reservoir needs to be changed. It may also be required in the rare event of performing a dye study to check catheter patency.

Calculating the initial priming dose

Formulae to calculate the initial pump and catheter priming dose and subsequent changes in drug concentrations need to be obtained from the pump system's manufacturers. In addition, they can advise on simple checks that can be performed to reduce the potential for error. For example, with the Medtronic systems, the initial priming dose should never be more than 0.5 ml or half of the solution concentration: for example, the maximum priming dose for 1000 μg/ml baclofen solution would be less than 500 μg.

The duration time for the priming dose can be calculated and set to ensure that the person can be closely monitored for this period, as this is a potential time for overdose to occur: for example, with the Medtronic systems, this can be set to run over 20 minutes. One safety mechanism is to programme the priming dose to occur in recovery, where anaesthetists are readily available to intervene if breathing difficulties occur. This enables the priming dose to be completed and the daily treatment dose commenced by the time the person is transferred back to the ward (see Appendix 8 for ward nursing care plans).

Calculating the initial daily dose

If the trial dose produces a clinical benefit of 6–8 hours, the initial daily treatment dose is calculated as:

> twice the most effective trial dose = the total dose delivered over 24 hours

For example, if following 25 μg the person's goal was partially achieved and the effect lasted 6 hours yet with 50 μg the goal was achieved and the effect lasted for 7 hours, the initial treatment dose would be 100 μg in 24 hours.

If the person has a positive effect for longer than 8 hours, the initial daily treatment dose is calculated as:

> the most effective trial dose = the total initial daily dose over 24 hours

For example, if a person achieved their goal following 25 μg for a period of 8 hours and following 50 μg for 12 hours, the initial dose would be 50 μg/day.

Clearly, if the aim is to preserve an individual's walking ability, a more cautious dose may be commenced, such as the daily treatment dose not exceeding the most effective trial dose.

Commencing dose titration

Over the first few days, the intrathecal dose can be titrated following discussion with the individual and feedback from members of the multidisciplinary team. Oral anti-spasticity medication doses may be titrated slowly downwards or remain unchanged until the person starts to feel an impact from the ITB on their spasticity and spasms. Often, the oral titration will not start until the person is an outpatient regularly visiting the refill clinic. Once the individual has been discharged and has returned to their normal daily activities, a truer picture of the impact of the ITB on their spasticity and spasms and how this is affecting their lifestyle can be appreciated, allowing the doses of both ITB and oral drugs to be titrated accordingly.

Changes to the ITB dose are made cautiously to reduce the risk of overdose; in addition, when titrating dosages in ambulant individuals, care is needed, as only small changes can have a profound effect on function. A good rule of thumb is to titrate at intervals of no more than 20%, but usually around 10% and even at increments of only 5% in ambulant individuals (Figure 7.5).

Discharge preparation

The individual's responsibility

At least one person – normally the person with the pump, but it can be a family member or carer – needs to take responsibility for the implanted pump system. This requires:

- commitment to attend for refills
- ongoing monitoring of effect on spasticity
- ongoing observation for signs of overdose (Table 7.2) and underdose, which can be characterised by persisting signs of spasticity such as stiff lower limbs, spasms and clonus
- awareness of the alarm systems and ability to take appropriate action to obtain medical assistance in both emergency and urgent situations (Table 7.4)

Figure 7.5

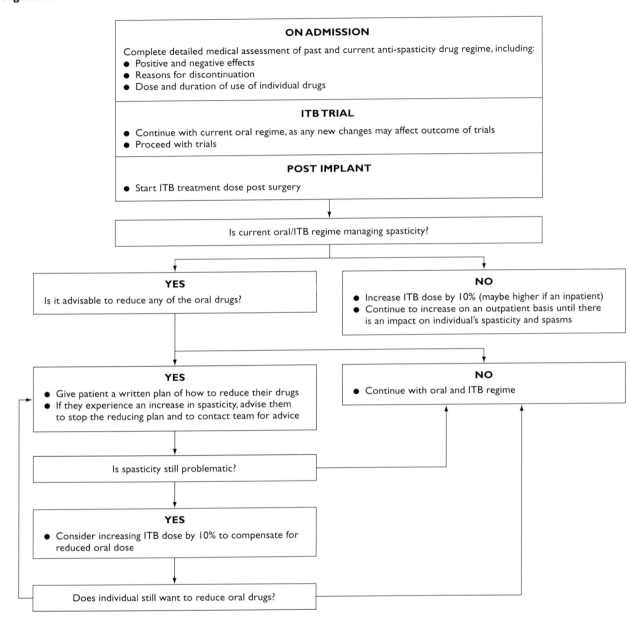

Titration of anti-spasticity drugs with the introduction of intrathecal baclofen (ITB)

Most electronic pumps have an inbuilt alarm system that will activate if the battery depletes, the pump malfunctions or the reservoir is low. The reservoir alarm can be set to activate before the reservoir is empty, ensuring that there is no break in treatment while an urgent refill appointment is organised. It is advisable that the reservoir volume alarm dates be monitored and appointments for refills arranged prior to these. In our service, this organisation and monitoring is a key responsibility of the nurse specialist. Some pumps can be programmed to give a demonstration of how the alarm may sound if activated; this is useful to demonstrate to individuals and their families prior to discharge. Often the alarms are of fairly low volume and are mainly heard by people during the night when background noise is minimal.

Table 7.4 When to seek medical assistance in an emergency or urgently in people with a baclofen pump

Emergency

Inform your close family and friends (plus work colleagues if you wish) to contact the emergency services (in the UK, telephone 999) if you ever show signs of:

- Difficulty breathing
- Being drowsy and are difficult to rouse
- Marked weakness in your legs

Urgent

Contact your specialist nurse or refill centre if:

- You hear an alarm
- There is a gradual or sudden change in your spasticity

Remember to monitor for the emergence of trigger factors, which may aggravate your spasticity, such as:

- Bladder and bowel problems
- Skin changes such as blisters or red or broken skin areas
- Any infections
- Tight clothing or splints

Liaising with community teams

Following the initial outpatient assessment clinic, all relevant healthcare professionals involved in the individual's care are sent a copy of the clinic report. Telephone contact is also made early in the process, often before admission, allowing plans for the admission, discharge and follow-up to be discussed, and if needed written information on ITB can be provided.

Prior to the individual's discharge, the outcomes of the trials and ongoing plans are discussed with the key people involved; often this includes the general practitioner (GP), district nurse, physiotherapist and wheelchair seating service. If a pump is implanted, a discharge pack that includes a written report plus details of the emergency contact procedure, alarm systems, potential side-effects and any pertinent articles is sent to members of the primary healthcare team.

Pump replacement

A database of implant dates and the expected year for replacement can allow a service to plan for and predict financial commitments on a yearly basis.

As the dates for replacement approach, individuals are reminded to inform the team of any changes in the level of their spasticity, as in our experience they may notice subtle changes before the pump low-battery alarm is activated.

Once it is thought the battery may be depleting, planning for pump replacement needs to be commenced. It is not clear how long the battery will continue to work before stopping altogether. Medtronic suggest that it may continue to function for 2–4 weeks, but they advise that a replacement be organised as soon as possible (Medtronic, personal communication). In our experience, pumps have lasted longer than this. However, if the individual's symptoms become unmanageable at home, an emergency admission may be required; if necessary, oral baclofen can be commenced during this time.

Replacement pump surgery

Providing that the catheter is patent, it is not replaced during surgery, leaving just the pump with the integral battery to be renewed. The reservoir is filled, but as the catheter is not replaced, a priming dose is not required. The normal treatment dose is prescribed and can be commenced as soon as possible, usually in recovery. A nursing care plan for pump replacement is detailed in Appendix 8.

It should, however, be noted that some baclofen can be lost during the surgery when the catheter and new pump are connected. It is not safe practice to routinely deliver a priming dose to account for this, as it is impossible to calculate the exact amount of baclofen lost. However, if it is clear to the surgeon that more than 0.5 ml of fluid was lost from the catheter during surgery and it is now filled with cerebrospinal fluid (CSF), a standard priming dose as when implanting a new pump can be given. Caution is needed when doing this, as there is a risk of overdose; however, failure to do it could lead to a gap in treatment until the catheter is filled – for those individuals on a low dose, this can be for several days.

Providing a 24-hour helpline for individuals and teams in the community

The number of people who are selected for ITB therapy is significant, but remains low in the overall population of any GP or community team's workload. It is therefore essential that adequate support to aid the safe delivery of ITB therapy be available. We have therefore developed a 24-hour hospital-based contact service, the details of which are given to the person with the pump, any family or carers involved, as well as their GP and community teams (Table 7.5).

Ongoing refill and follow-up

The pump design requires the reservoir to be refilled regularly; this is routinely done in an outpatient setting. At the NHNN, a neurologist and a specialist nurse hold ITB follow-up clinics jointly. At each clinic appointment, a spasticity management review is completed, the pump is refilled (a refill protocol is detailed in Appendix 12), dose adjustments are made and any further education with regard to tone management is discussed. Input from other therapists is accessed as necessary. Once an ITB pump is in place and the dose has been stabilised, the aim is to reduce, and possibly stop, other anti-spasticity agents, although this titration needs to be done judiciously, with appropriate increases in the dose of ITB as required. Outpatient dose titrations, whether increases or decreases, should rarely exceed 10% of the total daily dose due to the possibility of inducing side-effects (Figure 7.5).

The individual will often be the best judge of their spasticity management, and many will keep a diary or other notes on their progress for discussion in the clinic. In particular, whether the initial goal identified as part of the implantation process has been achieved will form an important part of the clinic review and will guide any further adjustments to either oral medication or the intrathecal dose. The length of time needed to reach an optimal therapeutic dose is extremely variable and is an ongoing process according to the clinical status of the person. Often, it requires liaison with members of the primary healthcare team and/or outpatient therapists to enable an individual's spasticity management and function to be maximised.

Frequently, individuals will have other medical issues that they would like to discuss in the clinic. In many cases, these can be related directly to the management of their spasticity (e.g. constipation or urinary incontinence): the clinicians need to decide whether they have the necessary skills to deal with these issues or whether referral to other specialists is indicated.

Troubleshooting

Problems may occur out of hours: therefore it is useful to have guidelines accessible for on-call medical teams. We have found the following sections useful to include in our protocol.

Treatment of overdose

Overdose (Table 7.2) is the most serious problem that can occur, and if the person is not already an inpatient, an emergency admission may be indicated. It is most likely to occur during the trial stage or following the refilling or reprogramming of a pump.

It is essential before treatment of an overdose to be sure that the person is indeed experiencing an overdose of baclofen and there is no other cause for toxicity. For instance, one person thought she was overdosing on ITB as her lower limbs had become very 'floppy', but on closer questioning this symptom coincided with her local neurologist starting her on gabapentin to treat her severe exacerbation of trigeminal neuralgia.

The treatment of baclofen overdose clearly depends on the degree of signs and symptoms. Priority should be placed on respiratory support, with intubation and mechanical ventilation being commenced if necessary.

No specific baclofen antagonist is available; however, there are reports of physostigmine given intravenously being useful in aiding reversal of mild central nervous system effects such as drowsiness and respiratory depression[23] (although other authors have

Table 7.5 24-hour support service for intrathecal baclofen therapy

- Between 08:30 and 17:00 Monday to Friday, the spasticity specialist nurses triage calls
- Between 17:00 and 08:30 and at weekends, the nurse in charge of the dedicated ward will triage calls. This involves the nurse taking the following information and then liaising with the neurologist on call:

1. Name
2. Contact telephone number
3. Reason for calling
4. Has their spasticity improved or deteriorated
5. Date last seen by a member of the spasticity team
6. Have they any other symptoms that may be aggravating their spasticity (e.g. urinary infection, retention, constipation or broken skin areas)

reported its failure to help in acute overdose[10]). Physostigmine should only be given in consultation with an anaesthetist. If it is given, a total dose of 1–2 mg may be administered intravenously over 5–10 minutes. Repeated doses of 1 mg may be administered at 30–60-minute intervals in an attempt to maintain adequate respiration in the absence of immediate facilities for respiratory support. Physostigmine is classified as an anticholinesterase that may be useful in the treatment of severe central anticholinergic toxicity. Its use should be reserved for serious situations because of potentially serious side-effects, which include bradycardia, cardiac conduction disturbances and convulsions.[23,24] Atropine sulphate should be readily available to treat bradycardia if necessary. For large overdoses, CSF withdrawal can be considered; this involves removing 30–50 ml of CSF via a lumbar puncture to reduce the baclofen load.

During the acute management of an overdose, the pump can be reprogrammed to give a lower dose of baclofen, or if necessary it may be stopped. The pump can be stopped by two methods:

- the reservoir of the pump can be emptied
- the pump can be turned off using the programmer

When stopping a pump, caution should be taken and close observations performed as seizures, tachycardia, hypotension, pyrexia, pruritis, rebound spasticity and decreased consciousness have all been associated with rapid withdrawal of baclofen.[25,26] Acute withdrawal syndromes have also been reported as progressing rapidly on to profound muscle rigidity, rhabdomyolysis, brain injury and even death.[27] These authors suggest that such a situation may be treated with oral baclofen, benzodiazepines or cyproheptadine while the reason for the acute withdrawal is established and rectified.[27]

Treatment of underdosage

The reason for the underdosage or increase in spasticity should be established before increasing the dose; for instance:

- Noxious stimuli may be exacerbating the spasticity. Treating these should be a priority.
- Deterioration in the underlying neurological condition may have led to increased spasticity.
- The pump reservoir may be empty or low on baclofen and the person may report a wearing-off

effect (some people have reported the latter as they approach the time for a refill).

- A catheter may be kinked, split or displaced.
- The pump may have a low battery.
- The pump may be malfunctioning.

Pump or catheter malfunction

Electronic pumps have alarms to alert if any problems are occurring. Whether or not an alarm is sounding, the electronic pump status can be checked by reading the pump with the programmer; this will identify the nature of any problem.

In addition, an ongoing regular check for pump efficiency can be made when the reservoir is refilled. The actual volume of baclofen removed from the reservoir can be checked against the expected amount: more or less than the expected volume (outside of accepted tolerances) could indicate an over- or underinfusing pump.

Using X-rays or scanners

There is unfortunately the potential for catheters to kink, split or become dislodged. A plain X-ray may be enough to determine the position of the pump and catheter, or a computed tomography (CT) scan may provide more detail. If a magnetic resonance imaging (MRI) scan is indicated, this will need to be discussed with a senior radiologist and the manufacturers to check the compatibility of the pump and the MRI scanner. The following points may also need to be considered:

1. Due to the pump, limited-SAR (specific absorption rate) scans may be necessary to limit the rise in tissue temperature adjacent to the pump. This unfortunately increases scanning time such that a normally routine scan may take up to 2 hours. As it is extremely important that the person lie completely still during the scan, a general anaesthetic may be required. The need for limited-SAR scans should be discussed with the radiologist.

2. Due to potential movement of the pump within the magnetic field, it is not recommended that ≥2.0 Tesla scanners are used.

3. If a Medtronic electronic pump is used, the magnetic field of the MRI scanner will stop the motor of the pump for the duration of the scan: this will mean that the person will not receive any

baclofen for that period of time. Whether they can be without the drug for this amount of time or they require oral baclofen cover needs to be decided.

4. The area around the pump on the scans will be distorted: this may limit interpretation. The radiologist will need specific details about the pump, to enable the amount of interference to be minimised.

5. The pump status needs to be ascertained using the programmer before and after the MRI scan to check that it is continuing to function appropriately.

Radiopaque dye study

Alternatively, if the pump has a catheter access port (Figure 7.2), a radiopaque dye study can be performed to check the patency of the catheter. This procedure can identify whether baclofen is leaking from the catheter at any point along its trajectory. This procedure normally requires an inpatient admission. The catheter is emptied of baclofen via the catheter access port; radiopaque dye is then inserted and its movement along the catheter is tracked via X-ray, during which any deviations in its course can be observed. It is important to ensure that the catheter has been emptied: otherwise a bolus of baclofen can be delivered with the dye, which could lead to an overdose.

Displaced pumps

Some pumps can become displaced, especially with individuals who gain weight post pump insertion.[28] It is not unusual for individuals whose frequent spasms are reduced or eradicated following pump insertion to gain weight; this may be due to reduced energy requirements. In the extreme, pumps can turn or flip over, thus preventing the reservoir from being refilled.[29] Manual or surgical manipulation may be necessary to enable repositioning.

Summary

ITB therapy can be a very effective management strategy for people with severe lower-limb spasticity and spasms; however, for some, the work involved is too great for the gains they will achieve. For those with severe, complex spasticity, intrathecal phenol may be a further option.

INTRATHECAL PHENOL THERAPY

The successful use of intrathecal phenol (IP) to reduce pain and spasticity was first reported in the 1950s;[30–32] however, due to the inherent destructive nature of the therapy, it was never completely accepted into the routine care of people with severe spasticity,[33] despite further reports of benefit from clinicians over the years.[34,35] In recent times, however, it has been recognised that a relatively small group of patients exist with severe, troublesome and often painful spasticity who cannot be effectively managed despite extensive physical and medical management programmes and who are not appropriate for ITB therapy or where symptoms are no longer managed by ITB. If these individuals are carefully assessed and appropriately selected, IP has been found to be a highly effective and well-tolerated treatment in the management of severe spasticity and associated pain.[36,37]

In the earlier studies, complications such as bladder and bowel incontinence, limb weakness, and painful paraesthesia were highlighted, although it was not clear if these complications resolved or persisted.[38,39] Another potential problem with IP therapy was the recognition that the beneficial effects may diminish over time, with pain and spasms returning.[40–42] This reoccurrence of symptoms is still well recognised, although IP should not be thought of as a temporary measure, as permanent impairment may still occur.[43] In our experience, this wearing-off phenomenon can necessitate repeat injections to maintain an effect, although the need for these may plateau after four or five injections over a timespan of approximately 2 years. The wearing-off is thought to be due to regenerating axons eventually re-innervating the motor endplates of the nerves.

Mode of action

Phenol is a neurolytic chemical that when injected peripherally or intrathecally causes coagulation of nervous tissue and denaturing of proteins, which leads to cell damage, axonal degeneration and indiscriminate destruction of motor and sensory nerves.[44] Injecting phenol with glycerol limits the dispersal into the CSF and nerve tissue, resulting in a relatively neuroselective effect, which can be further enhanced by specific positioning of the patient during and after the intrathecal injection, enabling motor nerve roots to be targeted while limiting the effect on sensory nerves (Figures 7.6 and 7.7).[37] Various concentrations and volumes of phenol solution have been reported to be useful. However, one study has noted that injecting smaller volumes of phenol in glycerol minimised the extent of side-effects; the concentration of phenol used was 5% and the volume injected ranged from 1.5 ml to 2.5 ml. The most prominent side-effect was transient changes in bowel function that lasted for a period of 4–6 weeks post injection.[37]

Outcomes of IP treatment

Spasticity, spasms and associated pain can be dramatically reduced or eradicated by IP therapy. This can lead to improved positioning, comfort and ease of carrying out personal care either for the individual or for their carers.

Figure 7.6

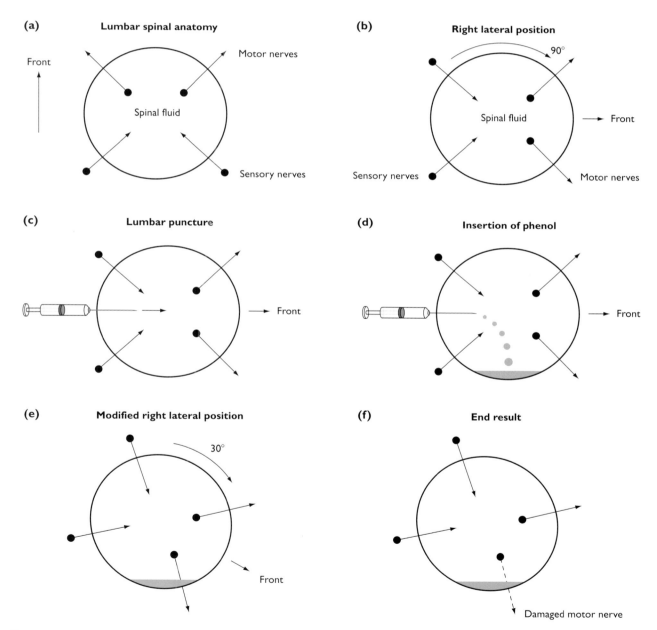

Diagrammatic representation of the intrathecal phenol injection process

Figure 7.7

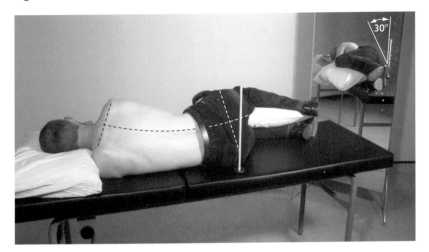

Modified lateral position with 30° pronation, used for intrathecal phenol injections. Reproduced with permission from Jarrett L, Nandi P, Thompson AJ. Managing severe lower limb spasticity in multiple sclerosis: Does intrathecal phenol have a role? J Neurol Neurosurg Psychiatry 2002,73:705–9

Adverse effects of IP therapy

Side-effects of IP treatment can be subdivided according to when they occur.

Short-term side-effects

These may occur during or soon after the injection procedure, and include hypotension, and heart rate and rhythm disturbances secondary to sympathetic nerve blockade. Very rarely, respiratory depression can occur. Post procedure, the individual may experience a low-pressure headache secondary to CSF leakage.

Long-term side-effects

These include changes in muscle power, sensation, and sexual, bowel and bladder function (Table 7.6). In addition to sensory impairment causing numbness, some people may experience a change in sensation, with the appearance of dysaesthetic pain or alteration in the character of pre-existing pain; this is more common with peripheral chemical neurolysis (Chapter 6), but can occur with intrathecal injections.

Secondary effects

The impact on a person's spasticity and positioning can be dramatic: if their posture is changed significantly, this often will have consequences for their seating and lying positions. The individual is likely to need a seating review to accommodate the sudden change in posture and to prevent complications such as pressure sores developing. For these reasons,

it is imperative that IP treatment only be carried out following close liaison with the relevant seating specialists or involved physiotherapist and/or occupational therapist.

In view of the potential long-term effects of treatment, careful patient education and selection is clearly essential before considering IP treatment.

Table 7.6 Potential long-term side-effects of intrathecal phenol

- Bladder and/or bowel retention or incontinence

- Sexual changes relating to reduced sensation in the perineal area and erectile dysfunction

- Reduced lower-limb sensation

- Lower-limb weakness within the range of movement available (often this is limited by contractures)

- Deep-vein thrombosis (DVT): spasms can promote vascular flow, so some patients may be at risk of DVT if their spasms are significantly reduced

- Neuropathic pain is uncommon with a subarachnoid neurolytic block, but can be caused by partial destruction of the somatic nerve and subsequent regeneration. It manifests clinically as hyperaesthesia and dysaesthesia that may be worse than the original pain associated with the spasticity

- Reduced skin integrity secondary to changes in posture in sitting and lying, as well as the effects of reduced sensation

Patient selection

In view of the invasive nature of IP therapy, selection of appropriate candidates requires detailed assessment and education of the individual and their family and carers. Due to the destructive nature of IP therapy, it is important to review whether other treatment options, such as the use of oral or other intrathecal drugs, inpatient or outpatient therapy, or a multi-disciplinary rehabilitation programme, have been considered and either thought not to be suitable or found to be ineffective. Furthermore, the use of IP should only be considered when bladder and bowel function are already compromised and effective management strategies are in place, and where there is severe pre-existing motor loss[36] and reduced sensation in the lower limbs (Table 7.7). IP interrupts neural innervation – it does not affect existing changes to muscle properties or contractures that have become fixed: it is essential to ensure that patients and their family or carers understand this. A neurophysiotherapy assessment can ascertain whether further physical measures or specialist seating may be able to improve positioning, although this is not always easy to predict.

Table 7.7   Selection criteria for intrathecal phenol

- Severe lower limb spasticity affecting comfort, function and/or care

- Maximum tolerated doses of oral medication have been tried without therapeutic effect

- Therapy and nursing intervention are no longer able to sustain effective management

- Other treatment options such as botulinum toxin and intrathecal baclofen are considered unsuitable or are no longer having a sustained effect

- Bladder and bowel impairment is evident, but effective management strategies are in place

- The individual is responsive to trial of intrathecal anaesthetic

- The individual and carer(s) are aware of the nature of treatment, potential short-term effects (e.g. hypotension) and long-term effects (e.g. changes to lower-limb sensation and to sexual, bladder and bowel function)

- The individual, family, carer(s) and the team collaboratively formulate and agree a goal of treatment, which will have a positive effect on the individual's daily life

---

The decision and treatment process

The overall treatment process (Figure 7.8) occurs in five stages: pre clinic, spasticity assessment clinic, post-clinic education, inpatient admission, and outpatient follow-up and reviews.

Pre clinic

As soon as the referral letter is received, the process of assessment of the individual begins. The aim of the work before the actual clinic appointment is to extend the information gained from the referral letter, ensuring that time in the clinic can be maximised. Details are gathered from the individual or from professionals currently involved with them. The different perspectives are sought on the main problems relating to the person's spasticity and past and current interventions used. These discussions also allow the development of a list of professionals to communicate with post clinic to enable a coordinated approach to the management plan. An integrated care pathway (ICP) (Appendix 1) is an effective mechanism to facilitate documentation and completion of the pre-admission process.

Spasticity assessment clinic

Any information received is reviewed and developed during the spasticity clinic assessment and recorded on the ICP. The person and their family or carers are asked to share what difficulties they encounter with their spasticity and what treatments have been helpful or unhelpful in the past. During this assessment, the team will also carry out a brief physical examination. The assessment process is outlined in full in Chapter 2. If IP is thought to be a potential management option, the person, their family and/or their carers are given both verbal and written information about the process (Appendix 13) and time to ask any questions.

Due to the destructive nature of this treatment, it is vitally important that education be appropriately paced to ensure that the individual and/or their carers have enough time to assimilate what is being proposed. In our service, the clinical nurse specialist provides the education and negotiates the most effective way to maintain telephone communication with the individual or nominated contact. It is useful to agree a time to call to continue with the education and to confirm whether or not they wish to proceed. Some people are sure at the clinic that IP is an option that

Figure 7.8

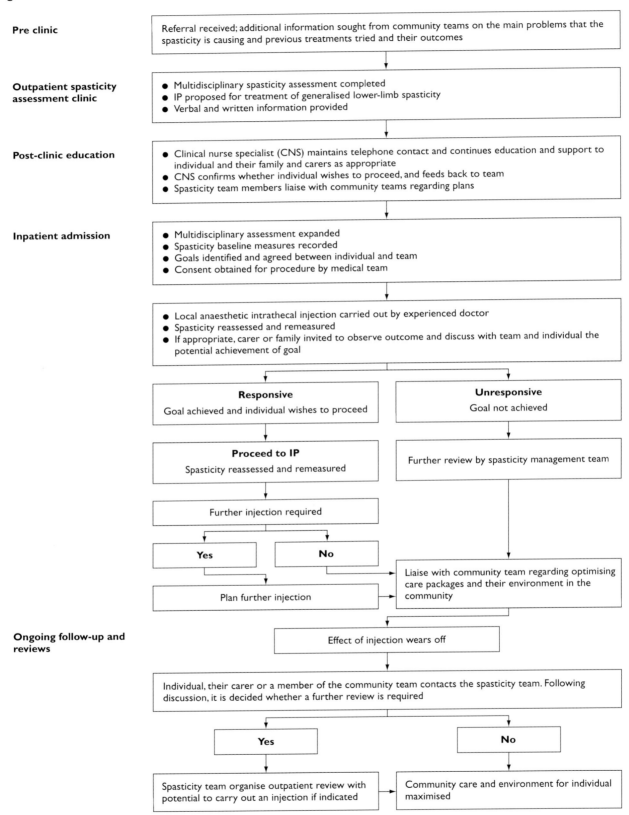

Intrathecal phenol (IP) treatment algorithm for managing severe lower-limb spasticity

they want to pursue; however, they are still contacted later to confirm and answer any questions or issues that may have arisen once they have had a chance to reflect on and assimilate both the verbal and written information.

Inpatient admission

On admission, the medical team completes a neurological assessment; the clinical nurse specialist and physiotherapist extend their assessment, complete a battery of measures (Appendix 2) and discuss a goal of treatment. Throughout this process, the education and information given to the individual and their families or carers about IP therapy is reviewed, with further opportunities for them to ask questions.

All of the information from the assessment is then considered by the spasticity team, the person and, if appropriate, their family or carer. The side for the trial injection (targeting the left or right leg) is then agreed and the overall goal of treatment is reviewed and finalised.

Engaging the person

A key management aim is to engage the individual throughout the assessment and treatment process. While this may seem obvious and a necessary aim of any treatment, individuals who are considering IP may have significant cognitive impairment. Enabling them to be involved in the process as far as they are able can be challenging, although often not insurmountable; strategies for doing this are outlined in Table 7.8. As the case example in Table 7.9 shows, time invested in doing this can be successful not only for working in partnership and developing therapeutic relationships between the individual and the professional, but also for uncovering what individuals are really hoping for as an outcome of the treatment. This ensures that expectations are known and can be discussed and debated with sensitivity. These issues can be difficult to address, but failure to do so can limit a person's understanding of what is hoped can be achieved – something that is essential when gaining informed consent. Open, honest dialogue on the expected outcomes, including what can and cannot be achieved, enables individuals, as far as they are able, to make informed choices about whether to proceed with treatment. Mostly, these discussions and decisions are made in partnership with the person, their family members or carers, and the team. However, in a

Table 7.8 Strategies to maximise a person's involvement in the decision-making process

- Establish the most effective method of communication from the individual or their family and carers

- For written information, consider the size of font required and what language would best convey the information to them? Would pictures help? Do they need you, a family member or a carer to read it to them? Consider providing multiple copies of the information, e.g. one copy each for the individual and their family and carers

- Repetition of information is normally required. Issues to consider include how quickly the person fatigues, how much information they can take in at one time, and whether an audio recording of the information would assist with providing repetition

- Be alert for when a person may be more receptive to information, and seize that opportunity. This requires paying ongoing attention to their level of engagement and flexibility with your time

- Use gentle probing questions during your interactions to establish if they comprehend what is occurring: e.g. Do you remember what we talked about yesterday? Have you got any questions from what we talked about earlier? This also enables you to assess whether they understand what is happening, or whether you need to repeat, emphasise or refine your education

- Consistency of staff involved in the information-giving not only builds a therapeutic rapport, but can also enable continuity in the dialogue, especially if the person responds best to short periods of education

situation where a person is unable to engage in the decision-making process, the focus for education will be their family or carers, although care should still be taken to explain to the individual the overall plan and to repeat the details of each stage of the process just before it occurs. If the person is unable to consent to the treatment and a member of their family or the team feel uneasy about the decision then the procedure should not go ahead.

The treatment procedure

There are two distinct phases in the treatment stage: the trial and the phenol injection.

Phase one: the trial

The anaesthetic bupivacaine acts by temporarily blocking nerve transmission by decreasing sodium

Table 7.9   Case example: Mabel

Mabel has multiple sclerosis; she has not walked for 5 years and has not been able to sit in her wheelchair for 18 months due to severe lower-limb spasticity and contractures. She was admitted for consideration of intrathecal phenol.

On admission, the doctor recorded that Mabel had severe cognitive impairment, and that her daughter had power of attorney and would be involved in the consent process. The doctor outlined to Mabel the reason for her admission. The clinical nurse specialist (CNS) and physiotherapist (PT) completed their assessment and outlined the treatment, its procedure and what it could and could not achieve. The goal of treatment was to try to enable Mabel to be seated in her wheelchair. At the end of this first day, the consultant reviewed Mabel, summarised the plan and reiterated the potential outcomes, and the goal of treatment was agreed.

When the CNS and PT were carrying out the measures on the next day, the CNS asked what Mabel wanted from the injection, she replied: 'To have straight legs and walk again.'

The CNS and PT gently discussed with Mabel how long it had been since she had walked, why she had possibly stopped being able to walk, why the injection would not make her walk, but what it could achieve. Mabel stopped engaging, refused eye contact, and tears ran down her face. This was painful and challenging for the CNS and PT; it was tempting at this point to collude with Mabel and use statements such as 'Who knows, perhaps you will walk again', when deep down both the CNS and PT knew that this would be extremely unlikely.

Over the next 2 days, the CNS spent significant periods of time with Mabel, discussing with her and her daughter what the treatment could and couldn't do. Mabel remained aloof from the CNS, and would not maintain eye contact and said very little. During the interactions, Mabel's hopes were acknowledged, as was how difficult it must be coming to terms with not being able to walk. The CNS shared how she and the rest of the team wanted to be honest with Mabel, which meant they would be truthful and clear about the aims of the treatment, ensuring that Mabel knew what the treatment could and could not do.

How Mabel was reacting was shared with the team; as each team member interacted with her, they were careful to remain consistent with information and not to build up any false hopes.

On day three, Mabel appeared brighter and more confident – she was smiling and maintaining eye contact. The CNS acknowledged this, and Mabel replied:

'You know that trial injection you keep going on about. Well I want to see what it could do for me, but I think it may hurt so I would like some pain killers before I go for the injection.'

Following the trial, Mabel went on to confirm that she did want to have the intrathecal phenol injections as it would help her use her wheelchair again so that she could visit her grandchildren.

---

channel permeability. The trial consists of injecting bupivacaine into the intrathecal space to produce a targeted, short-acting anaesthesia in order to ascertain whether or not the person's spasticity, spasms and/or pain could be managed more effectively with the longer-acting phenol injection. This trial allows the patient to temporarily experience the likely effect of having the phenol injection, and can assist them in deciding whether to proceed.

The trial injection procedure is outlined in Table 7.10. Side-effects can occur during the trial phase, but these are temporary. Hypotension can be a particular risk, and patients need to be carefully and closely observed during and after the procedure (nursing care

plans and a pre-injection checklist can be found in Appendix 14).

Both the local anaesthetic trial and the phenol will only have an effect on the neural component of tone and not on any biomechanical changes intrinsic to the muscles or soft tissues. One of the values of performing a local anaesthetic trial is the opportunity to remeasure and assess whether there are any contractures, which may limit the achievement of the goal. This enables the team to predict more clearly what the effects of the phenol may be to the person and their family. It is not uncommon for individuals and their families or carers to hope that the treatment will result in legs that can be straightened; the trial

Table 7.10   The injection guidelines

- It is advisable that intravenous access be obtained prior to the injection in case intravenous fluids or other drugs are required to maintain perfusion

- The side and level to be treated are confirmed and the patient is positioned lying on the targeted side. For example, if the right hip flexors are to be targeted then the patient will be positioned on their right side and the injection will be inserted at L2/3

- It is vital there be communication between the professionals carrying out the assessments and the medical specialist carrying out the injection to ensure that the correct area is targeted

- An expert medical practitioner who has been trained in the giving of intrathecal medication performs a lumbar puncture. A larger-gauge needle (e.g. size 18) will be needed to inject the phenol in glycerol as it is viscous

- In some situations the use of X-ray guidance to position the spinal needle may be required

- The solution is injected and the patient's position is checked by the injector. Repositioning may be required at this time to give some pronation, such as through the use of a wedge in order to target the motor nerves (Figures 7.6 and 7.7)

- The patient is maintained in this position after the trial injection for 5 minutes and following the phenol injection for 20 minutes

- The patient's blood pressure is recorded at least every 5 minutes for 30 minutes post procedure, and a specialist nurse observes them constantly for at least 1 hour

therefore allows them to appreciate the extent of any contractures and avoids any false hopes from the phenol injections.

The trial itself is an important part of the education process for the person, as even the best verbal and written education cannot surpass actually experiencing the injection process and its potential outcome and, together with the team, predicting how it may positively impact on daily life.

Phase two: the phenol injections

If the trial injection is successful, and the person wishes to go ahead, the phenol injections are planned. The process of the injection is the same as the trial except that a larger spinal needle (e.g. 18-gauge) may

be required, as the phenol is more viscous (Table 7.10). Typically, patients require both lower limbs to be targeted, and will therefore need two phenol injections; these are performed on separate days, ideally 24 hours apart to minimise any risk of short-term side-effects such as autonomic dysfunction. The outcome measures are repeated after the final treatment.

Outpatient follow-up and reviews

The outcomes of the treatment are fed back to the community teams and follow-up plans are confirmed. People who undergo IP therapy tend to have complex disabilities, and it can be difficult for them to travel to and from hospital on a regular basis. To limit the number of journeys and minimise disruption to often-detailed care packages, in our service, the community team commonly take responsibility for assessing the ongoing effect of the phenol and whether further injections may be necessary. If further treatment is required, the person or the community team can liaise with the hospital team and the repeat injections can be organised to be done on a half-day basis rather than necessitating a further hospital admission.

CONCLUSIONS

With careful patient selection and involvement of the individual in the decision-making and trial process, intrathecal therapies can be an effective management strategy for people with severe lower-limb spasticity and spasms.

For ITB to be used effectively requires a multidisciplinary infrastructure to work with the person with spasticity, not only to enable appropriate selection, education and assessment, but also to safely manage the trials, implant, ongoing review and dose titration. Strategies and mechanisms to support individuals to deal with emergency and urgent queries also need to be clearly defined. The commitment from the individual for the ongoing successful management of ITB cannot be overestimated, and developing therapeutic relationships between the team and the person is paramount to its success throughout the years of treatment.

The use of IP can also lead to positive outcomes, without the long-term follow-up issues that ITB entails or the side-effects often experienced in such individuals when on large doses of oral medication.

To maximise the outcomes fully of either intrathecal therapy, as with any intervention, there needs to be effective liaison between secondary and primary care, with clear negotiation of responsibilities for ongoing review.

Intrathecal therapies, in particular, are interventions where it is essential that the opportunity of working in partnership between the individual and professionals across the hospital and community interface be maximised.

REFERENCES

1. Penn RD, Kroin JS. Continuous intrathecal baclofen for severe spasticity. Lancet 1985;2:125–7.

2. Albright A, Cervi A, Singletary J. Intrathecal baclofen for spasticity in cerebral palsy. JAMA 1991;265:1418–422.

3. Meythaler JM, McCary A, Hadley M. Prospective assessment of continuous intrathecal infusion of baclofen for spasticity caused by acquired brain injury: a preliminary report. J Neurosurg 1997;87:415–19.

4. Penn RD, Davoy SM, Corcos D et al. Intrathecal baclofen for severe spinal spasticity. N Eng J Med 1988;320:1517–21.

5. Loubser PG, Narayan RK, Sandin KJ et al. Continuous infusion of intrathecal baclofen: long-term effects on spasticity in spinal cord injury. Paraplegia 1991;29:48–64.

6. Becker R, Benes L, Sure U et al. Intrathecal baclofen alleviates autonomic dysfunction in severe brain injury. J Clin Neurosci 2000;7:316–19.

7. Jarrett L, Leary SM, Porter B et al. Managing spasticity in people with multiple sclerosis. A goal orientated approach to intrathecal baclofen therapy. Int J MS Care 2001;3:2–11.

8. Meythaler JM, Guin-Renfroe S, Hadley MN. Continuously infused intrathecal baclofen for spastic/dystonic hemiplegia: a preliminary report. Am J Phys Med 1999;78:247–58.

9. Meythaler JM, Guin-Renfroe S, Brunner RC, Hadley MN. Intrathecal baclofen for spastic hypertonia from stroke. Stroke 2001;32:2099–109.

10. Coffey RJ, Cahill D, Steers W et al. Intrathecal baclofen for intractable spasticity of spinal origin: results of a long-term multicenter study. J Neurosurg 1993;78,226–32.

11. Ochs G, Strupper A, Meyerson BA et al. Intrathecal baclofen for long-term treatment of spasticity: a multicentre study. J Neurol Neurosurg Psychiatry 1989;52:933–9.

12. Zahavi A, Geertzen JHB, Middel B et al. Long term effect (more than five years) of intrathecal baclofen on impairment, disability and quality of life in patients with severe spasticity of spinal origin. J Neurol Neurosurg Psychiatry 2004;75:1553–7.

13. Leary SM, Gilpin P, Lockley L et al. Intrathecal baclofen therapy improves functional intelligibility of speech in cerebral palsy. Clin Rehabil 2006;in press.

14. Francois B, Vacher P, Roustan J et al. Intrathecal baclofen after traumatic brain injury: early treatment using a new technique to prevent spasticity. J Trauma 2001;50:158–61.

15. Fox S, Krnjevic K, Morris ME et al. Action of baclofen on mammalian synaptic transmission. Neuroscience 1978;3:495–515.

16. Davies J. Selective depression of synaptic excitation in cat spinal neurones by baclofen: an iontophoretic study. Br J Pharmacol 1981;72:373–84.

17. Davidoff RA, Sears ES. The effects of Lioresal on synaptic activity in the isolated spinal cord. Neurology 1974;24:957–63.

18. Becker WJ, Harris CJ, Long ML et al. Long term intrathecal baclofen therapy in patients with intractable spasticity. Can J Neurol Sci 1995;22:208–17.

19. Zierski J, Muller H, Dralle D, Wurdinger T. Implanted pump systems for treatment of spasticity. Acta Neurochir Suppl 1988;43:94–9.

20. Lioresal Data Sheet. Lioresal Intrathecal baclofen Injection. Minneapolis: Medtronic, 1996.

21. Delhaas EM, Verhagen J. Pregnancy in a quadriplegic patient treated with continuous intrathecal baclofen infusion to manage her severe spasticity: Case report, Paraplegia 1992;30:527–8.

22. Engrand N, Van de Perre P, Vilain G, Benhamou D. Intrathecal baclofen for severe tetanus in a pregnant woman. Eur J Anaesthesiol 2001;8:261–3.

23. Muller-Schwefe G, Penn RD. Physostigmine in the treatment of intrathecal baclofen overdose. J Neurosurg 1989;71:273–5.

24. Lazorthes Y, Sallerin-Caute B, Verdie JC et al. Chronic intrathecal baclofen for control of severe spasticity. J Neurosurg 1990;72:393–402.

25. Meythaler JM, Steers WD, Tuel SM et al. Continuous intrathecal baclofen in spinal cord spasticity. Am J Phys Med Rehabil 1992;71:321–7.

26. Coffey RJ, Edgar TS, Franscisco GE et al. Abrupt withdrawal from intrathecal baclofen: recognition and management of a potentially life-threatening syndrome. Arch Phys Med Rehabil 2002;83:735–41.

27. Meythaler JM, Roper JF, Brunner RC. Cyproheptadine for intrathecal baclofen withdrawal. Arch Phys Med Rehabil 2003;84:638–42.

28. Porter B. A review of intrathecal baclofen on the management of spasticity. Br J Nurs 1997;6:253–62.

29. Gianino J, York M, Paice J. Intrathecal Drug Therapy for Spasticity and Pain. London: Springer-Verlag, 1996.

30. Maher RM. Relief of pain in incurable cancer. Lancet 1955;1:18–20.

31. Kelly RE, Gautier-Smith PC. Intrathecal phenol in the treatment of reflex spasms and spasticity. Lancet 1959;2:102–5.

32. Nathan PW. Intrathecal phenol to relieve spasticity in paraplegia. Lancet 1959;2:1099–102.

33. Davis R. Spasticity following spinal cord injury. Clin Orthop Relat Res 1975;112:66–75.

34. Browne RA, Catton DV. The use of intrathecal phenol for muscle spasms in multiple sclerosis: a description of two cases. Can Anaesth Soc J 1975;22:208–18.

35. Scott BA, Weinstein Z, Chiteman R, Pulliam MW. Intrathecal phenol and glycerin in metrizamide for treatment of intractable spasms in paraplegia. Case report. J Neurosurg 1985;631:125–7.

36. Williams JE, Shepherd J, Williams K. Rediscovery of an old technique to treat severe spasticity: intrathecal phenol. Br J Ther Rehabil 1995;2:209–10.

37. Jarrett L, Nandi P, Thompson AJ. Managing severe lower limb spasticity in multiple sclerosis: Does intrathecal phenol have a role? J Neurol Neurosurg Psychiatry 2002;73:705–9.

38. Nathan PW, Scott TG. Intrathecal phenol for intractable pain. Lancet 1958;1:76–80.

39. Wood KM. The use of phenol as a neurolytic agent: a review. Pain 1978;5:205–29.

40. Lourie H, Vanasupa P. Comments on the use of intraspinal phenol- pantopaque for relief of pain and spasticity. J Neurosurg 1963;20:60–3.

41. Hansebout R, Cosgrove JBR. Effects of intrathecal phenol in man: a histological study. Neurology 1966;6:277–82.

42. Nathan PW. Treatment of spasticity with perineural injections of phenol. Dev Med Child Neurol 1969;311:384.

43. Gelber DA, Jozefczyk PB. The management of spasticity in multiple sclerosis. Int J MS Care 1999;1:1–15.

44. Bonica JJ. Neurolytic blockade and hypophysectomy. In: Bonica JJ (ed). The Management of Pain, 2nd edn. London: Lea & Febiger, 1990:1980–3.

45. Ashworth B. Preliminary trial of carisoprodal in multiple sclerosis. Practitioner 1964;192:540–2.

Chapter 8

Setting up a service

Valerie L Stevenson, Louise Jarrett and Louise J Lockley

There is no right or wrong way to set up or design a service, and many simply grow ad hoc from ongoing clinical commitments or research studies. However, particularly in today's health services, it is usually necessary to present a business case to support appropriate funding for clinical teams and departments that are often already overstretched. The thought of writing a business case can be daunting, but it is often an excellent way of clarifying the precise nature of the proposed service development. Appropriate spasticity services will differ according to the needs of the local population and available resources. Depending on where the services are – for example whether in primary or secondary care – the key drivers for the service development and proposed members of the team involved may differ. However, there are several universal considerations that deserve attention when planning a new service (Table 8.1).

ROLES OF THE TEAM

When considering the members of a spasticity team, it is necessary to understand what each professional can uniquely offer. Undoubtedly, roles will overlap, but it is helpful to understand the specialised core skills of each profession in order to assess what they could offer the service. An outline of the key skills and roles of a potential core team is given in the following section. The development of detailed job descriptions and competency frameworks can be advantageous in guiding and developing team members (an

example of a set of specific competencies for a nurse specialist in intrathecal baclofen is included in Appendix 9).

Doctor

The doctor should:

- understand the underlying neurological condition, including prognosis, natural history, associated features and possible complications
- identify abnormal features or unexpected changes that may suggest an alternative cause or second pathology
- be experienced in history-taking and neurological examination
- be competent in the prescribing and use of pharmacological interventions, including oral medication, botulinum toxin and intrathecal drug therapies

Nurse

The nurse should:

- educate the individual to manage their own spasticity, involving family members and carers if appropriate
- manage cutaneous and visceral stimuli
- advise on posture, moving and handling
- manage psychosocial issues
- consider the impact of spasticity and its treatment on role, employment and social activities

Table 8.1   Considerations for business case planning

• Needs of local population	• Liaise with local purchasers, providers and users: e.g. community teams, local rehabilitation units and voluntary or patient groups. Should the service be located in primary or secondary care?
• What will the service look like to enable needs to be met?	• Will this be an outpatient or community service offering focal treatments, or will complex spasticity be considered, including inpatient assessment, rehabilitation or intrathecal therapies?
• Who will refer into the service?	• Need to consider contingency plans for under- or oversubscription to the service
• Who is needed to make up the core team? E.g. doctor, physiotherapist, nurse, occupational therapist or seating services	• Need to consider individual roles and competencies required for the service, and how team members will be managed
• Is there access to link services such as orthotics, functional electrical stimulation, splinting, rehabilitation and therapy?	• Integrating with and complementing established services will strengthening the case for the new service
• Funding in the short and long term for posts, equipment, ongoing drug costs and surgical needs	• Will the new service impact on old services, allowing reconfiguring of posts, or will the new service generate income sufficient to cover running costs? Consider industry or charitable sources of funding, bearing in mind these are usually for a defined time period, often focusing on set-up
• Secretarial and administrative support	• Often a forgotten factor, but vital to the smooth running of any service
• Systems for monitoring the safety of the service	• Appropriate clinical guidelines and protocols are essential and enable auditing
• Systems for monitoring the effectiveness of interventions	• Accurate assessment and use of appropriate outcome measures needed to detect clinical change
• How will the value of the service be assessed?	• Consider feedback mechanisms from users, referrers and service managers
• Provision of education to users of the service and promotion of their self-management	• Appropriate and timely use of patient information sources are needed
• Ongoing education of team members	• Consider training to achieve necessary competencies
• How will research and development be incorporated into the service	• These elements need to be built into the job descriptions of all team members, alongside clinical and management responsibilities. A dynamic innovative team with a vision is more likely to succeed in realising their proposed business case development while also enhancing service provision and developing knowledge

- work with individuals, their families or carers to appreciate the nature of invasive treatments and potential impact on their daily lives
- monitor the ongoing accuracy of guidelines and protocols in relation to safe delivery of services, particularly with invasive treatments

Physiotherapist

The physiotherapist should:

- explore the potential for movement patterns and functional ability to be enhanced
- identify trigger factors of spasticity and spasms related to posture and movement
- consider the relative contributions of neural and biomechanical components to spasticity and limit further soft tissue shortening and loss of function
- identify underlying muscle weakness and the impact on function

Occupational therapist

The occupational therapist should:

- assess and if necessary provide splints to preserve soft tissue length and promote function
- assess posture and seating, if necessary liaising with specialist seating services
- assess the impact of spasticity on roles and function
- consider access to work, home and community environments

Other disciplines, although not necessarily part of the core team, clearly have expertise to offer in other areas, and can be liaised with as needed. These include rehabilitation physicians, neurologists, neurophysiologists, speech and language therapists, orthotists, social workers, continence advisors, and psychologists. Access to a skilled neurophysiologist may be particularly valuable when considering the assessment of focal spasticity with electromyography (EMG) to facilitate accurate muscle localisation for botulinum toxin therapy.

In addition to the above roles, one team member will need to be responsible for the overall day-to-day running of the service. This ensures smooth running of the service, limits duplications and provides leadership to junior members of the team. The leadership role does not necessarily need to be discipline-specific – it may fall to the individual who has been in the service longest or perhaps to the person with the most

dedicated time for the service. It is important that this role be reflected in their job description due to the time constraints and responsibility that it entails. In our team, this role is performed by one of our nurse specialists.

GROWING YOUR SERVICE

It is of course important to be realistic with service developments and appreciate that they grow over time, often with stepwise developments secondary to successful business case planning, research proposals, and external drivers such as government initiatives or the launch of new therapeutic options. It is very unusual for a comprehensive service to be developed de novo, with new personnel all arriving at once. This process is illustrated by our service at the National Hospital for Neurology and Neurosurgery (NHNN), London, which has developed to its current status over the last 10 years (Table 8.2). At each stage of development, plans are already being formulated to produce the next business case to support the subsequent period of growth.

All services will come under pressure – whether from internal drivers to increase activity or reduce waiting times, from central government targets, from media attention or from the voluntary sector (e.g. campaigns for the use of cannabis-based medication). These, however, can be viewed as opportunities to further develop and enhance services through timely business planning. In addition to these pressures, it is also possible to seize opportunities from research or audit studies.

RESEARCH AND DEVELOPMENT

It is extremely important to allow time for research and development in the job descriptions of all of the team members. This not only provides time to maintain databases but also allows for the development of patient-focused services, including information provision, and for strategic development. Involvement in research studies promotes knowledge and skill development, as well as providing opportunities for service expansion through dedicated research-funded posts. Often, by translating such studies directly into clinical practice, service development can be enhanced. The pathway in Table 8.2 demonstrates how evidence from research and expert groups was used to inform

Table 8.2 Development of the spasticity service at the National Hospital for Neurology and Neurosurgery (NHNN), London

Research and development	Pathway to integration into spasticity service
1. Increasing awareness of intrathecal baclofen (ITB) therapy through published research. The neurology team explored the use of treatment at NHNN	• Clinical governance issues were raised, in particular with regard to the safety of administering ITB and effective education of patient and ward staff[8] • A joint business case was produced between neurology and rehabilitation services to develop the infrastructure for running an ITB service • Role for part-time ITB nurse practitioner was developed. This post had lead responsibility for the ITB service, involving the development of protocols and education tools to ensure safe and effective service delivery
2. Research trial of botulinum toxin for spasticity, involving consultant neurologist, neurophysiologist, senior physiotherapist, and medical and physiotherapy research fellows[1]	• After research was completed, focal spasticity management expertise was incorporated into a neurophysiotherapy clinical specialist role. Focal treatment clinics continued within the clinical service
3. Standards were developed for multiple sclerosis (MS) services between the Multiple Sclerosis Society of Great Britain and Northern Ireland and NHNN[9]	• NHNN did not meet standards, so a business case was submitted to improve the service provided • An MS nurse post was designed, incorporating the part-time ITB post. This post maintained and developed the protocols and standard of service delivered, developed the advanced nursing role in refilling/reprogramming pumps, and provided education to medical and therapy colleagues on all aspects of the ITB service • A generalised spasticity assessment clinic was developed, incorporating both focal and generalised treatment options. The clinicians involved were a consultant neurologist, a clinical neurophysiotherapy specialist and an MS nurse specialist. There was additional input from a neurophysiologist when required
4. Disease-modifying drugs for people with MS became more widely available	• Demand on the MS service increased at all stages of disease evolution. There was difficulty maintaining the ITB service within the MS population and recognition that the spasticity service needed to reach beyond the MS population. A business case was submitted to expand and distinguish between services • A full-time ITB nurse practitioner role was developed
5. The ITB service was reviewed.[2] The referral rate to the spasticity outpatient assessment clinic increased, with a corresponding rise in inpatient work	• The ITB nurse practitioner role expanded to incorporate all spasticity-related nursing issues. The post title became spasticity management nurse specialist • A business case was developed for a part-time physiotherapy clinical specialist dedicated to spasticity management
6. The intrathecal phenol (IP) service was reviewed[3] 7. The ITB and IP service continued to expand	• A business case was developed for a second specialist nurse

Research and development	Pathway to integration into spasticity service
8. With a further increase in outpatient assessment referrals, the waiting list became unmanageable	• A business case was submitted to increase neurology, physiotherapy and secretarial input to the service

Current team

• Lead consultant neurologist responsible for overall clinical spasticity service, including assessment clinics, ITB and IP inpatient and outpatient services (3 sessions/week)

• Consultant neurologist responsible for focal spasticity assessment and treatment clinics (2 sessions/month)

• Senior nurse specialist (full-time) responsible for day-to-day running of service. Key clinical areas: spasticity assessment clinics and IP service lead

• Nurse specialist (full-time): ITB service lead

• Physiotherapy clinical specialist (half-time) responsible for assessment clinics and inpatient and outpatient services

• Senior 1 physiotherapist (full-time) responsible for focal spasticity assessment clinics and supporting inpatient and outpatient services

• Secretarial and administrative support (full-time)

and develop the NHNN spasticity service over a time period of approximately 10 years. This included a research study looking at the effectiveness of botulinum toxin,[1] which not only added to the growing literature but also contributed to the development of the present clinic that combines the assessment and treatment of both focal and generalised spasticity (Table 8.2). In a similar way, retrospective reviews of data collected from patients receiving both intrathecal phenol and intrathecal baclofen allowed us to detail the effectiveness and side-effect profile of these interventions. This information guided future consent protocols and encouraged us to develop both services further.[2,3]

IMPROVING SERVICES THROUGH AUDIT AND INTEGRATED CARE PATHWAYS

Although business planning is instrumental in enabling substantial changes to service provision, the use of audit can streamline and improve existing processes. The audit process can be facilitated by defining the ideal patient journey into an integrated care pathway (ICP). This is a document that describes a process within health and social care and that collects variations between planned and actual care.

The concept of ICPs in health and social care grew from the recognition of the importance of critical path and process mapping methodology used in industry since the 1950s. In the early 1990s, the UK National Health Service (NHS) funded a patient-focused initiative to support organisational change. This resulted in the investigation and development of concepts such as pathways that were already in use in the USA. By 1994, the ICP had evolved in the UK into clinician-led and -driven documents with patients and locally agreed best practice at their heart. In response to the demand for a coordinated ICP users group, the National Pathways User Group (later renamed the National Pathway Association) was set up in 1994. This continued until 2002, when the National Electronic Library for Health (NeLH) Pathways Database was launched to enable the free sharing of ICPs and ICP Projects across the UK.[4]

WHAT IS AN ICP?

An ICP is defined by the NeLH is as follows:[4]

An ICP is a document that describes the process for a discrete element of service. It sets out anticipated, evidence-based, best practice and outcomes that are locally agreed and that reflect a patient-centred, multidisciplinary, multiagency approach. The ICP document is structured around the unique ICP variance tracking tool. When used with a patient/client, the ICP document becomes all or part of the contemporaneous patient/client record, where both completed activities and outcomes, and variations between planned and actual activities and outcomes, are recorded at the point of delivery.

Important areas highlighted by this definition are to ensure that the ICP forms the clinical record and is not a repetition of information recorded elsewhere, and that it is based on locally or nationally agreed best practice for the specific patient group. Although ICPs may contain protocols and guidelines, they do not act as decision-making aids. Integral to the concept of the ICP is a mechanism for recording variations or deviations from planned care: these variances can be used for future auditing of service delivery and patient care. The incorporation of such clinical indicators and measurable goals ensures that the audit process is embedded within the care pathway. When used appropriately, ICPs offer the potential to deliver a coherent plan of care and treatment with less fragmentation and duplication, while aiding coordination and communication between social, primary and secondary care.[5,6]

Guidelines to aid in the development of ICPs can be found on the NeLH website.[4]

AUDIT AND ICP DEVELOPMENT – A WORKING EXAMPLE

The following example details the growth of our pre-admission ICP and subsequent service development through audit.

Audit

Following the audit of outpatient attendances to the NHNN Spasticity Assessment Clinic, several problems with the service were identified:

1. There was an increasing number of referrals to manage in the same amount of clinic time.
2. Clinic time was not being used optimally, due to:
   - insufficient information from the referrer regarding previous spasticity management strategies and community nursing and therapy input
   - follow-up therapy not prearranged for potential botulinum toxin therapy candidates, necessitating a second clinic appointment for the injections once the therapy was in place, thus using two appointments instead of one

- an unknown level of anticoagulation for those patients taking warfarin, necessitating a second appointment for botulinum toxin injections
- incomplete assessment for patients with severe communication difficulties when no carer/advocate attended the clinic with them
- information regarding the patient being documented in several places: medical, physiotherapy and nursing notes
- appointments unable to be filled at short notice if cancellations occurred

ICP development

To address these problems and thus improve the efficiency of the clinic and the quality of service provided, an ICP was developed over 1 year by the spasticity team and the Trust Governance Department. The team's opinion, along with available literature of best practice in spasticity management, experience of the clinic and the RCP National Guidelines for the use of botulinum toxin in the management of spasticity in adults[7] were all used to develop the ICP.

The aims of the ICP were to:

- improve the efficiency of the service from receipt of the referral to assessment and through to follow-up
- reduce the number of unfilled appointments
- reduce the need for extra appointments
- minimise repetition of multidisciplinary team (MDT) records

The document was developed and refined over the year through regular review and audit by the spasticity team (Appendix 1).

The ICP is split into three sections:

1. *Pre-clinic information collection.* This includes details such as referral dates, waiting time and variances for clinic attendance. It also enables screening for those on warfarin (and thus facilitates stabilisation of anticoagulation levels) and organisation of physiotherapy for those patients referred for botulinum toxin injections. Screening of the medical notes is included if the team feel that appropriate details of previous interventions for spasticity management and information on

the community teams involved would be valuable for the assessment. The community teams are contacted to gain further information.

2. *Multidisciplinary assessment.* Details of the assessment are recorded during the clinic by the different team members, including plans of action and variances. The ICP is not stapled, enabling different pages to be completed simultaneously by different team members during the clinic to maximise efficiency.

3. *Post-clinic action.* This section includes details of actions agreed and taken, along with any variances in the pathway.

Ongoing assessment

To assess the impact of the ICP on the specific problems identified in the service, several key issues were audited at 1 year:

1. Were those patients who were assessed as suitable for botulinum toxin able to be injected at the same clinic visit?
   - Was physiotherapy follow-up organised before the clinic for those people referred for botulinum toxin injections?
   - Were patients on warfarin who were potential botulinum toxin therapy candidates identified before clinic, and if so, were anticoagulation levels optimised before the clinic?
2. Was information gathered before the clinic, and where was the information gained from?
3. Was the documentation collaborative?

Results in these three areas were very encouraging:

1. All patients who were identified as being suitable for botulinum toxin had their injections in the first clinic visit, with no second appointments being needed. All had physiotherapy organised before the clinic, with the first therapy appointment arranged for 7–14 days after the clinic. All were screened for warfarin use, and if identified had anticoagulation levels suitable for injection on the day of the clinic. This reduced the need for second appointments for the injections, thus allowing more patients to be seen.
2. Information was sought for all patients referred. The information was gained from a variety of sources, including the individual, family members

or carers, local community teams, district nurses, and other hospital departments, including therapy services. The information was most useful where patients were unable to communicate issues relating to their spasticity management.

3. Nursing, physiotherapy and neurophysiology notes were all in one document, although medical notes were also recorded concurrently. The ICP had also facilitated a joint MDT report compiled on each patient using all of the information from the ICP and the medical notes, which is routinely sent to the GP, hospital consultants, community teams and the patient.

The use of the ICP, particularly through the pre-clinic screening, clearly increased the efficiency of the spasticity clinic and ensured that a single visit to the clinic is sufficient to complete an assessment and instigate management strategies for the majority of patients. It also serves to alert the community teams to the referral.

By identifying those people taking warfarin who have been referred for botulinum toxin injections, it also provides a risk management strategy to avoid wasted clinic visits or the possibility of injecting while at a level of anticoagulation deemed unsafe (an international normalised ratio (INR) above 2.5 in our clinic).[1]

Acquisition of information before the clinic has enabled the specialist team to tailor assessment to individual needs and maximise the use of clinic time to benefit the patient. This information has proved invaluable where there are communication difficulties and has facilitated carers to attend the clinic when appropriate.

Lessons learnt

Although undoubtedly the introduction of an ICP to the outpatient spasticity service has improved the efficiency of the service, the gathering of pre-clinic information obviously takes time and this needs to be allowed for when planning service development.

This ICP took 1 year to develop, and in order that its effectiveness be maintained, it needs to be reviewed regularly though ongoing audit. Ensuring that ICP data are entered onto an electronic database facilitates this ongoing audit and variance analysis. Maintenance of the ICP database is clearly also time-consuming – something that was reflected in our latest business case, which highlighted the need for dedicated secretarial support to the clinical team.

CONCLUSIONS

Careful consideration is necessary when setting up a new service or developing an existing one. Although business planning is often perceived as a time-consuming chore it is an excellent way to clarify how an ideal service should look for the specific population concerned. Through close liaison with existing services and consideration of necessary competencies and skillsets for team members, a valued clinical service can be created. The use of ICPs and regular audit will ensure that this is of the highest quality for users and referrers, while incorporating research and development will continue to expand knowledge and drive the service forward.

REFERENCES

1. Richardson D, Sheean G, Werring D et al. Evaluating the role of botulinum toxin in the management of focal hypertonia in adults. J Neurol Neurosurg Psychiatry 2000;69:499–506.

2. Jarrett L, Leary SM, Porter B et al. Managing spasticity in people with multiple sclerosis. A goal orientated approach to intrathecal baclofen therapy. Int J MS Care 2001;3:2–11.

3. Jarrett L, Nandi P, Thompson AJ. Managing severe lower limb spasticity in multiple sclerosis: does intrathecal phenol have a role. J Neurol Neurosurg Psychiatry 2002;73:705–9.

4. About Integrated Care Pathways (ICPs). http://libraries.nelh.nhs.uk/pathways/aboutICPs.asp

5. Kitchiner D, Davidson C, Bundred P. Integrated care pathways: effective tools for continuous evaluation of clinical practice. J Eval Clin Pract 1996;2:65–9.

6. Lowe C. Care pathways: have they a place in 'the new National Health Service'? J Nurs Manag 1998;6:303–6.

7. Royal College of Physicians. Guidelines for the Use of Botulinum Toxin (BTX) in the Management of Spasticity in Adults. London: Royal College of Physicians, 2002.

8. Porter BA. A review of intrathecal baclofen on the management of spasticity. Br J Nurs 1997;6:253–62.

9. MS Society. Standards of Health Care for People with MS, 1997. www.mssociety.org.uk/what_is_ms/publications_shop/devel_ms_hlthc.html. Accessed 17.02.06.

Section II

Appendix 1

Spasticity clinic integrated care pathway

Confidential Patient Information

Patient name (or attach ID label)	
Hospital/NHS number	
Date of birth	
Address	
Home telephone number	
Work telephone number	
Mobile telephone number	
Allergies	

Staff present at assessment in clinic	
Consultant neurologist	
Nurse specialist	
Neuro physiotherapist	
Visitors	

Professional and Contact Details	Professional and Contact Details
Name	Name
Title	Title
Address	Address
Telephone number	Telephone number
Fax number	Fax number
Name	Name
Title	Title
Address	Address

Pre-Clinic Information	
Referral date:	
Referral source: Name	Medical referral letter required: Yes No If yes, Date referral requested / / . Date referral received / / .
Neurologist/Rehabilitation Physician/General Physician/Physiotherapist/Nurse:	
Diagnosis:	GP:
Neurologist:	If botulinum toxin, are they On warfarin Yes No Contact : GP Anticoagulation clinic
Reason for referral	Last INR level: _____ Date: / / (needs to be below 2.5)
Spasticity:	Discuss level with medical team: Yes No Action taken:
Botulinum toxin:	Post-clinic therapy arranged: Yes No
Anticipated clinic date: Clinic date appointment sent for: Actual clinic attended:	
Variance	
Secretary to send Botulinum Toxin Form with MDT Report post clinic: Yes No	

Acceptable abbreviations for use in this pathway. Muscle abbreviation list on page 122

CNS	Clinical nurse specialist		Add	Adductor
S/N	Staff nurse		Flex	Flexion
SpR	Specialist registrar		Ext	Extension
PT	Physiotherapist		UL	Upper limb
OT	Occupational therapy		LL	Lower limb
Pt	Patient		Rt	Right
ICP	Integrated care pathway		Lt	Left
NHNN	National Hospital for Neurology and Neurosurgery		DIP	Distal interphalangeal joint
ITB	Intrathecal baclofen		PIP	Proximal interphalangeal joint
BT	Botulinum toxin		MCP	Metacarpalphalangeal joint
IP	Intrathecal phenol		MTP	Metatarsalphalangeal joint
ISC	Intemittent self-catheterisation		EMG	Electromyogram

ALL STAFF SIGNING FOR CARE IN THIS ICP MUST RECORD BELOW DETAILS OF THEIR FULL NAME, POSITION AND SAMPLE SIGNATURE

FULL NAME – Please Print	POSITION	SIGNATURE	INITIAL	CONTACT DETAILS

Pre-Clinic Information

Date and time	Person contacted	Outcome of contact	Signature

Spasticity Management ICP: **Out-Patient Clinic – Physical Assessment**

Posture	Tone	Selective movement	Function

Analysis and summary

Therapist:

Spasticity management ICP Out-patient clinic – spasticity assessment (see later for BT assessment)	Patient's name Hospital number Date of birth	**Date**	

Diagnosis:

Current medication	Please comment on dose, route, times and any side-effects experienced
Other medication used in the past for spasticity: Why did they stop taking it (ineffective, not tolerated, other reason?)	
Primary difficulty: Is it attributed to spasticity: Yes No	Severity rating out of 10
Other difficulties related to spasticity:	
Spasticity	Please comment on site and severity of spasticity
Not needing to be assessed ☐	

Clonus	**Please comment whether spontaneous**
Not needing to be assessed ☐	
Spasms	**Please comment on which muscles, extensors or flexors, severity, pain, frequency and duration**
Not needing to be assessed ☐	
Pain	**Please comment on presence, severity and management. Indicate if pain has been getting worse, better or remains the same**
Not needing to be assessed ☐	
Sleep patterns	**Please comment on disturbances, positions and quality**
Bed mobility	**Please comment on how much, type of mattress used**
Not needing to be assessed ☐	
Bladder	**Please comment on current management**
Not needing to be assessed ☐	
Bowel	**Please comment on current management**
Not needing to be assessed ☐	
Skin	**Please comment on the presence of pressure ulcers and the ability to relieve pressure, change position and sensation and any aids used (Waterlow Tool, see later)**
Not needing to be assessed ☐	
Waterlow Score =	**Not needing to be assessed ☐**
Mobility	**Please comment on outdoor, indoor, aids, speed and distance**
Not needing to be assessed ☐	
Toilet/bath/shower transfers	**Please comment on ability and aids required. Indicate if this has been getting worse, better or remains the same**
Not needing to be assessed ☐	
Transfers	**Please comment on car, bed, chair, level of independence and assistance required**
Not needing to be assessed ☐	
Wheelchair	**Please comment on posture, position, type and make of chair and cushion**
Not needing to be assessed ☐	
Previous therapy and nursing input	**Please comment on physiotherapy, OT, seating assessments, and nursing advice. Ensure details of time, date and location of treatment obtained, including names, addresses and contact details.**
Options discussed with patient	**Make a note of the type of information discussed. For example, oral medication, dosage, therapy input, BT, ITB, IP, seating assessments, splinting etc.**

Written information provided:		
Spasticity management:	Intrathecal baclofen:	
Drug company information – tizanidine:	Intrathecal phenol:	
Exercise and stretching:		
Action to be taken: (Please include details of who will implement the action)		
Refer for therapy at **NHNN**		
Refer for local therapy input		
Change oral medication		
Admission for further assessment		
Admission for intrathecal baclofen trial		
Admission for intrathecal phenol		
Referral for seating assessment		
Referral to another discipline		
Consider **IT** option and liaise with **Nurse** Specialist Spasticity Management		
No action needed except **MDT** letter back to referrer and existing services.		
Assessment signed on behalf of the team Name (please print) _____ Signature: _____ Designation: _____ Bleep Number: _____		

Spasticity Management ICP Botulinum Toxin Assessment					
Informed consent	YES			NO	
Information leaflet given	YES			NO	

Main problem relating to spasticity:

Baseline measures:

Analysis of problem/clinical reason

Goal:

Goal information sheet given to patient/carer

Recommendations:

Follow-up plans:

Action needed by team:	Date action completed

Variance   No variance

Assessment signed on behalf of the team

Name (please print) _____ Signature: _____

Designation: _____ Bleep Number: _____

Muscle Abbreviations:
Acceptable abbreviations used in this pathway

Upper Limb

Delt	Deltoid	ECR	Extensor carpi radialis
Lat d	Latissimus dorsi	ECU	Extensor carpi ulnaris
Pec Maj	Pectoralis major	E dig	Extensor digitorum
Pec Min	Pectoralis minor	E dig min	Extensor digiti minimi
Biceps	Biceps brachii	EPL	Extensor pollicis longus
Brach	Brachialis	EPB	Extensor pollicis brevis
BR	Brachioradialis	Add poll	Adductor pollicis
FCR	Flexor carpi radialis	Abd poll	Abductor pollicis brevis
FCU	Flexor carpi ulnaris	Lumb	Lumbricals
FDS	Flexor digitorum superficialis	Pron ter	Pronatus teres
FDP	Flexor digitorum profundus	Pron quad	Pronator quadratus
FPL	Flexor pollicis longus	Supin	Supinator
FPB	Flexor pollicis brevis		

Lower Limb

Add mag	Adductor magnus	Tib ant	Tibialis anterior
Add long	Adductor longus	Tib post	Tibialis posterior
Add brev	Adductor brevis	EDL	Extensor digitorum longus
Semi-m	Semi-membranosous	EHL	Extensor hallicus longus
Semi-t	Semi-tendinosus	Gastroc	Gastrocnemius
Biceps f	Biceps femoris	Soleus	Soleus
Psoas	Psoas major	FHL	Flexor hallicus longus
Iliac	Iliacus	FHB	Flexor hallicus brevis
		FDB	Flexor digitorum brevis

Botulinum Treatment		
Type of BT used		
Dilution	_____ Units/ _____ ml saline	
Muscle identification	Palpation / **EMG** / Stimulation	
Muscles Injected		
Muscle	**Left – units**	**Right – units**

Signature of injector:

Name (please print): _____ Signature: _____

Designation: _____ Bleep Number: _____

Clinic Summary				
Code	**ACTION**	**Date**	**Reason for variance and action taken (use codes)**	**Sign**
M1	Spasticity assessment completed			
M2	Baseline measures recorded			
M3	Treatment options discussed with patient			
M4	Action plan written			
M5	Post-clinic action completed			
M6	If applicable, botulinum toxin assessment completed			
M7	Informed consent obtained and signed			
M8	Patient given information leaflet and goal sheet			
M9	Patient aware of follow-up appointment			
M10	Post-clinic letters sent to secretary Date:			
M11	Letters signed, date:			
M12	Outcome form received:			
M13	Goal achieved: **Yes No**			
M14	Need for further BT identified			
M15	Action taken:			

Guidance Tools						

WATERLOW SCORE

Build/weight for height		Condition of pressure areas		Sex/Age		Special risks	
Average	0	**Visual Risk**		Male	1	Tissue malnutrition	
Above average	1			Female	2	(e.g. terminal cachexia)	8
Obese	2	Healthy	0			Cardiac failure	5
Below average	3	Tissue paper	1	14–49	1	Peripheral vascular disease	5
		Dry	1	50–64	2	Anaemia	2
Continence		Oedematous	1	65–74	3	Smoking	1
		Clammy (temp. up)	1	75–80	4		
Complete/catheterised	0	Discoloured	2	81+	5	Neurological deficit (active)	4–6
Occ. Incontinent (1/day)	2	Broken/spot	3			(e.g. diabetes, MS, CVA,	
Cath./incont. faeces	2			**Appetite**		motor/sensory, paraplegia)	4–6
Doubly incontinent	3	**Mobility**					
				Average	0	**Major surgery/trauma**	
		Fully	0	Poor	1		
		Restless	1	NG tube (for aspirate)	2	Orthopaedic – #NOF	5
		Apathetic/depressed	2	Fluids only	2	Below waist, spinal	5
		Restricted	3	NBM/anorexic	3	Op. table > 2 h	5
		Traction/bed rest	4				
		Chairbound	5			**Medication**	
						Steroids, cytotoxics, high-dose anti-inflammatory	4

Total Score Rating:
    10+ = patient at risk
    15+ = patient at high risk
    20+ = patient at very high risk

Ashworth Scale	
0	No increase in muscle tone
1	Slight increase in muscle tone, manifested by a catch and release or by minimal resistance at the end range of motion when the part is moved in flexion or extension/abduction or adduction
2	More marked increase in muscle tone through most of the range of movement, but the affected part moved easily
3	Considerable increase in muscle tone, passive movement difficult
4	Affected part is rigid in flexion and extension (adduction or abduction)

Post-clinic telephone calls			
Date and time	To whom	Comment	Signature

VARIANCE CODES

	Specific to spasticity management			
401	Patient not responding to telephone messages	417	Further nursing assessment needed
402	Patient not responding to letters	418	Transport did not arrive
403	Patient choice	419	Secretary not available
404	Patient refuses treatment	420	Neurology staff not available
405	Patient unable to communicate	421	Neurophysiology staff not available
406	Patient too unwell to travel	422	No community nurse involved
407	Fixed contracture	423	No community therapist involved
408	Patient too uncomfortable to participate	424	Community team failed to provide information
409	Muscle not actively contracting on EMG	425	Care home staff not available
410	Appointment delayed as patient in hospital	426	More detailed physiotherapy assessment needed outside clinic
411	Appointment delayed at patient's request	427	More detailed medical assessment needed outside clinic
412	Appointment delayed as unable to organise follow-up	428	INR level not suitable for injection
413	More detailed nursing assessment needed outside clinic	429	INR not known
414	Further discussion with local team needed	430	Information not checked pre-clinic
415	Further medical assessment needed	431	Waterlow recorded for potential inpatients only
416	Further physiotherapy assessment needed	432	Patient moved clinic due to waiting time targets for GP referrals

UCLH Trust VARIANCE CODES

	Patient condition			
001	Pyrexia	014	Wound infection
002	Nausea and/or vomiting	015	Chest infection /UTI
003	Pain not controlled	016	MRSA-positive
004	Wound bleeding/oozing	017	Other infection (Please state in notes)
005	Drain oozing/excessive drainage	018	Poor mobility
006	Hypertensive	019	Mobilising faster than expected
007	Hypotensive	020	Fatigue/sedation
008	Pressure area concern	021	Asleep
009	Poor urine output	022	Confused
010	Constipation	023	Communication problem
011	Low blood glucose	024	Other patient condition issue
012	High blood glucose	025	Deep-vein thrombosis
013	Catheter in situ	026	Pulmonary embolism

Staff/persons				
101	Medical staff decision	108	Physiotherapist not available
102	Medical staff not available	109	Family's decision
103	Nursing staff decision	110	Family unavailable
104	Nursing staff not available	111	Other clinician/AHP decision
105	Patient's decision	112	Other clinician/AHP not available
106	Patient not available	113	Other staff/person issue
107	Physiotherapist decision		
Departmental system			
201	Done/given previously	209	Nursing staff unavailable
202	Pharmacy delay	210	Medical staff unavailable
203	Trust patient transport delay	211	Physiotherapist unavailable
204	Laboratory delay	212	OT unavailable
205	X-ray delay	213	Bed unavailable in unit
206	Other departmental delay	214	Community care unavailable
207	Equipment unavailable	215	Other clinical staff unavailable
208	Weekend/out of department hours	216	Other departmental system issue
External system			
301	Bed unavailable in other hospital/unit	304	District/community nurse delay
302	Other hospital transport delay	305	Other community service delay
303	Social services delay	306	Other external system issue

(Additional space to record details of other professional contacts, pre-clinic information and for the assessment process should be inserted when adapting for use in specific service settings)

Appendix 2

Generalised spasticity outcome measures form

Name: **Date of Assessments:**
Hospital No.:   **Ax 1**   **Ax 2**   **Ax 3**   **Ax 4**

1. **Goniometry to measure range of passive movement** (Norkin and White 1985)
   - Position patient in supine where possible and record the resting angles at hip, knee and ankle with a goniometer. Note 0 is the neutral position of the joint
   - Record the full passive range available at each joint, i.e. knee range $20°-100°$, where $0°$ represents a straight or neutral hip or knee joints
   - Hip abduction is measured in crook lying with the hips and knees flexed and measurement taken from one bony prominence of the medial aspect of the knee to the other

Left Leg

Joint	Resting angle Ax1 Ax2 Ax3 Ax4	Full range available Ax1 Ax2 Ax3 Ax4	Comments
Hip flexion–extension			
Hip abduction–adduction			
Knee flexion–extension			
Ankle PF–DF			

Right Leg

Joint	Resting angle Ax1 Ax2 Ax3 Ax4	Full range available Ax1 Ax2 Ax3 Ax4	Comments
Hip flexion–extension			
Hip abduction–adduction			
Knee flexion–extension			
Ankle PF–DF			

2. Maximum distance between knees as measured during passive hip abduction
(Hyman 2000)

Measure the maximum distance between knee joint lines

	Ax 1	Ax 2	Ax 3	Ax 4
Distance in mm				

3. Ashworth scale (Ashworth 1964)

To standardise the measure, it is recommended to:
- Perform 3 passive movements only and score the resistance felt on the third movement
- The score is taken within the available range
- Move the limbs in the best alignment possible
- Regulate the speed by counting 1001, 1002, 1003

Resistance to:	Ax 1		Ax 2		Ax 3		Ax 4	
	L	R	L	R	L	R	L	R
Hip and knee flexion in supine								
Hip and knee extension in supine								
Hip abduction in crook lying								
Ankle dorsiflexion with knee extended								

Ashworth Scale

0 = **No increase in muscle tone**

1 = **Slight increase in tone giving a catch when the limb is moved**

2 = **More marked increase in tone but limb easily moved**

3 = **Considerable increase in tone – passive movement difficult**

4 = **Limb is rigid in flexion or extension, abduction or adduction**

4. Adductor tone rating (Snow 1990)

Measure in crook-lying:

0 = No increase in tone; 1 = Increase tone, hips easily abducted to 45° by one person; 2 = Hips abducted to 45° by one person with mild effort; 3 = Hips abducted to 45° by one person with moderate effort; 4 = Two people required to abduct the hips to 45°

	Ax 1	Ax 2	Ax 3	Ax 4
Rating				

5. Active range of movement (Norkin and White 1985)

Record the active range available using a goniometer:

	Ax 1	Ax 2	Ax 3	Ax 4
Hip flex–ext				
Hip abd–add				
Knee flex–ext				
Ankle PF–DF				

6. Spasm frequency scale (Penn 1988)

0 = No spasms
1 = Mild spasms induced by stimulation
2 = Infrequent spasms occurring less than once an hour
3 = Spasms occurring more than once per hour
4 = Spasms occurring more than 10 times per hour

Score	Ax 1	Ax 2	Ax 3	Ax 4
Left				
Right				

Description of spasms

- **Type at Ax 1:**
  Ax 2:
  Ax 3:
  Ax 4:

- **Triggers at Ax 1:**
  Ax 2:
  Ax 3:
  Ax 4:

7. Clonus and spasms score (self-report) (Smith 1994)

0 = Absent
1 = Provoked by painful stimuli only
2 = Provoked by touch, light pressure and/or occasionally spontaneous (5/day and/or <2/night)
3 = Provoked by passive movements (during physical therapy or nursing care) and/or frequently spontaneous (>5/day and/or 2/night)

Score	Ax 1	Ax 2	Ax 3	Ax 4
Left clonus				
Left spasm				
Right clonus				
Right spasm				

8. Numeric rating pain intensity scale (NRS) (Kremer 1978)

Ask the patient: On a scale of 0–10, in which 0 is no pain and 10 is the most severe pain you could possibly imagine, what would you give your pain at this moment?

	Ax 1	Ax 2	Ax 3	Ax 4
NRS (out of 10)				

9. Numeric rating scale for leg stiffness

Ask the patient: On a scale of 0–10, in which 0 is no stiffness and 10 is the most severe stiffness you could possibly imagine, what would you rate your leg stiffness at the moment?

	Ax 1	Ax 2	Ax 3	Ax 4
NRS (out of 10)				

10. Posture in seating score (record if predominantly a wheelchair user; if not, omit)

(A) Seating posture score
Please record 0 = yes, 1 = no (observe subject while sitting in the wheelchair and answer 0 or 1 to the four questions). Take the sum of the four questions and record in the 'total' box

	Ax 1	Ax 2	Ax 3	Ax 4
Are the feet well positioned on the footplates?				
Are the knees apart?				
Are the hips well aligned?				
Is the trunk posture symmetrical?				
Total				

(B) Baseline sitting tolerance score
Fit the subject into the most appropriate category and record the number. This score may only be applicable at initial assessment and on outpatient follow-up

0–1 hour = 4   1–2 hours = 3   2–6 hours = 2   6 hours = 1

	Ax 1	Ax 2	Ax 3
Score			

Initial Assessment Photo Date	Final Assessment Photo Date

11. Walking and falls scores

(A) Record the frequency of falls over the last month
This may only be applicable on initial assessment and follow-up appointments

0 = No falls   1 = 2–3 falls per week
2 = 5–6 falls per week   3 = Daily falls
4 = More than 1 fall per day

	Ax 1	Date	Ax 2	Date
Score				

(B) 10-metre timed walk (Wade 1987)

Date | **Date** | **Date** | **Date**
No. of steps = ... | No. of steps = ... | No. of steps = ... | No. of steps = ...
Time   = ... | Time   = ... | Time   = ... | Time   = ...
Aid used   = ... | Aid used   = ... | Aid used   = ... | Aid used   = ...

12. Overall comfort rating
Ask the patient how comfortable they have felt over the last 24 hours. Rate the level of comfort on a scale of 0–10: 0 = very comfortable; 10 = extremely uncomfortable.

	Ax 1	Ax 2	Ax 3	Ax 4
Rating (out of 10)				

13. Identify the main problem that is amenable to treatment
....
....
....

14. Goal agreed between the team and the patient and/or carer (related to the main problem identified)
....
....
....

Please circle achievement of the goal and date:

Ax 2   Date   Achieved   Not achieved
Ax 3   Date   Achieved   Not achieved
Ax 4   Date   Achieved   Not achieved

GUIDELINES FOR GONIOMETRY TO MEASURE HIP, KNEE AND ANKLE PASSIVE RANGE OF MOVEMENT*

Hip

- Measure in supine.
- Place the fulcrum of the goniometer over the lateral aspect of the hip joint using the greater trochanter of the femur as a reference.
- Align the proximal arm with the lateral midline of the pelvis.
- Align the distal arm with the lateral midline of the femur using the lateral condyle for reference.
- For the moderate to severe group of patients with spasticity, take a measure of the full passive range available, where 0° is the neutral position of the hip, i.e. 20°–120°. This would indicate a 20° flexion contracture.

Hip abduction

- As these patients tend to be unable to be positioned with hips and knees in a neutral position in supine, it is recommended that this measurement be performed in a crook-lying position with a tape measure rather than using a goniometer.

Knee

- Measure in supine with the knee extended.
- Centre the fulcrum of the goniometer over the lateral condyle of the femur, using the greater trochanter for reference.
- Align the distal arm with the lateral midline of the fibula, using the lateral malleolus and fibular head for reference.
- Measure the full passive range available from the neutral/straight-knee position, which will be 0°, i.e. 30°–140°. This would indicate a 30° flexion contracture.

Ankle

- Measure in supine with the knee in at least 30° of flexion and the foot in 0° of inversion and eversion.

* Adapted from Norkin CC, White DJ. Measurement of Joint Motion: A Guide to Goniometry. Philadelphia: FA Davis, 1985.

- Centre the fulcrum of the goniometer over the lateral aspect of the lateral malleolus.
- Align the proximal arm with the lateral midline of the fibula, using the head of the fibula for reference.
- Align the distal arm parallel to the 5th metatarsal.
- The starting position is 90° at the ankle, and this is recorded as 0° for the goniometry.
- Move the ankle into dorsiflexion and then into plantarflexion to record the full range available.
- To record, start with the plantarflexion angle, then to 0° and then to the dorsiflexion angle: e.g. 40°–0°–10°.

REFERENCES

Ashworth B. Preliminary trial of carisoprodal in multiple sclerosis. Practitioner 1964;192:540–2.

Hyman N, Barnes M, Bhakta B et al. Botulinum toxin (Dysport) treatment of hip adductor spasticity in multiple sclerosis: a prospective, randomised, double blind, placebo controlled, dose ranging study. J Neurol Neurosurg Psychiatry 2000;68:707–12.

Kremer E, Atkinson JH, Ignelzi RJ. Measurement of pain: patient preference does not confound pain measurement. Pain 1981;10:241–8.

Norkin CC, White DJ. Measurement of Joint Motion: A Guide to Goniometry. Philadelphia: FA Davis, 1985.

Penn RD, Savoy SM, Corcos D et al. Intrathecal baclofen for severe spinal spasticity. N Engl J Med 1989;320:1517–21.

Smith C, Birnbaum G, Carlter JL et al. Tizanidine treatment of spasticity caused by multiple sclerosis: results of a double-blind, placebo-controlled trial. US Tizanidine Study Group. Neurology 1994;44:S34–42.

Snow BJ, Tsui JKC, Bhatt MH et al. Treatment of spasticity with botulinum toxin: a double blind study. Ann Neurol 1990;28:512–15.

Wade DT, Wood VA, Heller A et al. Walking after stroke: measurement and recovery over the first three months. Scand J Rehab Med 1987;19:25–30.

Appendix 3

Managing your spasticity and spasms

What is spasticity?

Spasticity can be described as involuntary muscle stiffness. It can range from mild to severe and can change over time, often from day to day or hour to hour. Symptoms can be unpleasant, but sometimes spasticity can be helpful: if a person's legs are very weak, the stiffness that spasticity causes may actually help in transferring from bed to chair or even in walking. The key to successful management of spasticity is the individual, who needs to be aware of management strategies that they can incorporate into daily life.

Why does spasticity occur?

Nerve pathways connecting the brain, spinal cord and muscles work together to coordinate movements of the body. These pathways can be disrupted in neurological conditions such as stroke, multiple sclerosis, and head or spinal cord injury. This leads to loss of coordination and overactivity of muscles – so-called spasticity.

So what are the symptoms?

The main feature of spasticity is stiffness or increased resistance when attempting to move a limb or joint. Other features that may be associated with it include spasms, pain, weakness and clonus.

Stiffness/increased resistance to movement

Some people with spasticity describe that their muscles feel stiff and heavy and are difficult to move. In very severe cases, it can be very difficult to bend a limb at all. If a limb becomes fixed in one position, this is known as a contracture.

Your healthcare team may comment on the tone in your limbs. Muscle tone is described as the resistance felt when trying to move or stretch an arm or leg. Normal tone is when an individual is relaxed and the healthcare professional can bend and straighten the limb without difficulty. When spasticity is present, there is an increased resistance to the movement (an increase in tone).

Muscle stiffness and increased tone can also occur in an individual's trunk/body. Sometimes, individuals can have mixed symptoms. For example, their trunk/body may be weak or floppy, but their legs may be stiff and difficult to move. These mixed symptoms need careful management.

Spasms

Spasms can be described as sudden involuntary contractions of muscles that can make your arms, legs or body move in different ways: see for example Table 1.

Severe spasms may make your back arch off the bed or chair.

Table 1

Flexor spasms	The limb will bend upwards towards your body	
Extensor spasms	The limb will shoot out away from your body	
Adductor spasms	The limb will pull inwards towards your body. Commonly this can be when your thighs stay together and it is difficult to separate them	

Pain

Spasticity can be painful – but not always. If pain is present, it may be linked to spasms or stiff muscles or may be a consequence of altered sitting and lying positions.

Weakness

Despite a limb resisting movement (an increase in tone), the muscles may also be weak: this may increase the feeling of heaviness in arms or legs.

Clonus

This is a repetitive up-and-down movement, often of the feet. It may be observed as a constant tapping of a foot on wheelchair footplates.

Other symptoms associated with spasticity can include fatigue and loss of dexterity.

What problems can spasticity cause?

Spasticity and its associated features can affect all aspects of daily life. For instance, it may change the way you walk, transfer, sit in a chair, turn over in bed or carry out your care needs, it may affect your sexual activities, and it can affect your overall comfort and mood. Furthermore, persistent spasticity can lead to poor postures in lying and sitting, which can lead to pain, pressure sores or contractures (when a limb becomes fixed in one position). However, there are many steps that you can take to minimise the impact of spasticity on your daily life.

What can I do and who can help me?

Increasing your knowledge about spasticity and what triggers it can help you to manage it more effectively and prevent symptoms. Whether you have mild or severe symptoms, medical, physiotherapy, nursing and occupational therapy treatment, advice and education could help increase your understanding and management. The factors listed in Table 2 are particularly important, as they can aggravate spasticity and its associated features.

Available treatments

Physiotherapy

It is important to keep muscles, ligaments and joints as flexible as possible. Spasticity, spasms and weakness

Table 2

Aggravating factors	*Who can give management advice*
• Urinary infection or retention • Bowel impaction, constipation, infection • Red or broken skin/pressure areas • Ingrown toenails	• Sometimes you may notice that your spasticity is becoming harder to manage; it may be that a review of your bladder, bowel and skin care management techniques will improve the situation • Your GP, a nurse specialist, a continence advisor and/or a district nurse can give advice and assistance to effectively manage your bladder, bowels and skin
• Tight-fitting clothes or splints	• Simply loosening tight garments may help to relieve spasticity • If splints are causing discomfort or skin irritation then they will need reviewing by your orthotic or therapy services
• Pain • Infections	• Pain and infection will aggravate spasticity. If the source of the pain or infection can be located (e.g. a skin infection or an ingrown toenail), then treating this may help reduce your spasticity. Advice can be sought from your GP or district nurse
• Poor positioning in sitting, lying and standing: 	• A good position when lying, sitting or standing will help you manage your spasms and spasticity and prevent discomfort and contractures developing • For example, when in any chair, if possible sit with your hips and bottom at the back of the seat, with your knees and feet at right-angles • Putting weight through a spasm can reduce its intensity: for example, if you can do so safely, either stand or lean forward in your chair to transfer weight to reduce lower-limb spasms • A physiotherapist and/or occupational therapist will be able to advise on your sitting, lying, standing posture and possibly suggest exercises to help manage your spasticity • If necessary, your local wheelchair service can recommend a suitable wheelchair to optimise your management

can result in muscle shortening and joint stiffness, which in turn can aggravate spasticity and spasms. A physiotherapist can advise on how to maintain flexibility, and can teach specific stretches and ways of moving and positioning the body in order to prevent contractures.

As well as looking at the above measures to reduce spasticity, it is sometimes necessary to use medication to optimise management.

Oral medication

Baclofen

This is the most commonly prescribed medication for spasticity; it acts directly on nerve cells, mainly in the spinal cord, to decrease the excitability of the nerves and therefore reduces excessive muscle activity includ-

ing spasms. Most people do not experience side-effects, provided that the baclofen is started at low doses (often at 5–10 mg once or twice a day) and slowly increased, stopping at a dose that helps but does not cause any problems (maximum dose 40 mg three times a day). The effect of an oral baclofen dose can last between 4–6 hours, so it needs to be taken regularly to ensure adequate control of symptoms. Side-effects can include weakness, drowsiness and dizziness. Baclofen should not be greatly reduced or stopped suddenly without asking your doctor, as this can also cause side-effects.

Tizanidine

This also works on the central nervous system and needs to be introduced slowly to avoid side-effects (started at 2 mg a day and increased up to a maximum of 36 mg daily). It is claimed that tizanidine does not increase muscle weakness as much as baclofen, but this varies between individuals. When on this drug, your doctor will take blood samples regularly to ensure that it is not having any adverse effect on your liver function. Other side-effects can include drowsiness and dry mouth.

Diazepam and clonazepam

These drugs can be used alone or, more commonly, in combination with other drugs. Clonazepam is particularly useful taken at bedtime if spasms are a problem at night. The main side-effect is drowsiness, which is not a problem if either drug is taken at bedtime. Neither diazepam nor clonazepam should be stopped suddenly without asking your doctor.

Dantrolene

This is the only antispasmodic drug that works directly on the muscles rather than on the central nervous system. It can be used in combination with other drugs. Side-effects are unfortunately quite common: they include nausea, vomiting, diarrhoea and weakness. Rarely, dantrolene can cause liver problems: therefore, while you are on this drug, your doctor will regularly take blood samples to check that this is not a problem for you.

Gabapentin

This is a drug that is used to treat epilepsy and some types of pain. It also has some effect on spasticity and can be used in combination with other drugs; it is particularly useful if pain and spasticity coexist. Gabapentin is started at a low dose (300 mg per day) and increased up to a maximum of 1200 mg three times a day. It should not be stopped suddenly without discussing with your doctor. Side-effects include drowsiness, dizziness and blurred vision.

Key points in all drug treatments

Using drugs to assist you in managing your spasticity can be invaluable. To get the maximum benefit from your drugs you should work out the best time to take them that will help you carry out your activities during the day. For instance, if getting out of bed is difficult, have your drugs next to your bed, take them when you wake up and then wait 10–20 minutes before getting up.

What if the drugs don't help me?

If your management strategies, therapy input and oral drugs are not providing adequate relief then the following treatments may be considered.

Intramuscular botulinum toxin

This is a toxin that when injected into muscles causes them to become weak and less stiff. It can take 14 days for the full effect to occur. It is useful for small muscles, and must be used in conjunction with physiotherapy or occupational therapy. Often the injections can allow therapists and yourself to work with the muscle more effectively, to minimise the effects of the spasticity. Sometimes repeated injections are necessary.

Intrathecal baclofen therapy

When baclofen is taken orally as tablets, it has to build up in the bloodstream before it can reach the nerve cells in the spinal cord or brain to reduce the spasticity and spasms. Sometimes people cannot tolerate a high enough dose of oral baclofen to help their spasticity without getting side-effects.

Intrathecal baclofen therapy is another way of delivering baclofen. It delivers the drug directly onto the nerve cells in the spinal cord. In the short term, this can be done via a lumbar puncture, but if long-term treatment is required then an implantable pump can deliver it. The pump is surgically placed in the abdomen and a catheter delivers the baclofen into the intrathecal space (the space around the spinal cord within the spine). It uses much smaller amounts of baclofen to treat spasticity, reducing any side-effects that a person may have experienced when taking baclofen orally.

Intrathecal baclofen therapy is used to treat generalised lower-limb spasticity. It requires commitment from individuals not only during the trial and implant phase but also for the ongoing maintenance of regular pump refills and replacements.

Intrathecal phenol

Injecting phenol into the intrathecal space stops nerve conduction and can reduce lower-limb spasticity.

Repeat injections can be performed if required. Transient negative effects on the sensation in your legs, sexual function, bladder and bowel management can occur. However, if you already have effective management strategies in place (e.g. a suprapubic catheter) or use suppositories regularly, the use of intrathecal phenol may not cause you any further negative effects.

Surgery

Occasionally, your neurologist may recommend orthopaedic or neurosurgical procedures.

Useful telephone numbers

Hospital team

_____

Community team

_____

National helplines

_____

Appendix 4

Managing spasticity and spasms with exercise

What are spasticity, spasms and contractures?

Spasticity can be described as involuntary muscle stiffness. People with spasticity describe their muscles as feeling stiff, heavy and difficult to move.

Spasms can be described as sudden involuntary contractions of muscles. They can make your arms, legs or body move in different ways. For example:

- Flexor spasms will move a limb towards your body.
- Extensor spasms will move the limb away from your body.
- Adductor spasms will pull the limb inwards towards your body. Commonly, this can be when your thighs stay together and it is difficult to separate them.

Contractures are when a limb becomes fixed in one position. This occurs if spasticity and spasms persist, restricting movement and causing limbs to be held in set positions. This can lead to a loss of mobility in your joints and muscles, and in the long term a contracture can develop. Once a contracture develops, it is difficult to treat and change the position of the limb.

Clonus is a repetitive up-and-down movement, often of the feet. It may be observed as a constant tapping of a foot on wheelchair footplates.

Why is exercise important?

Regular exercise is very important not only in helping to reduce spasticity and spasms but also to prevent contractures. Even the smallest amount of exercise, either carried out by you or by a person helping you to move your limbs, will be beneficial. Movement and stretching help to keep muscles, joints and ligaments supple and flexible. There are different types of exercise, and a combination of stretching, strengthening and cardiovascular exercise is generally recommended. A physiotherapist can help you devise an individualised exercise programme that realistically fits into your daily life.

This leaflet concentrates mainly on stretches that you can carry out either on your own or with the help of another person. A physiotherapist can advise you which of these stretches would be suitable for you and how many times you would need to perform them each day. As well as carrying out the stretches, it is also important to try to change your position regularly – for example standing up or lying flat if you are sitting for long periods. Positioning aids such as a T-roll or pillows may be helpful if it is difficult for you to hold a position. Where possible, try to move each part of your body during the day.

Stretching exercises

All of these stretches are best performed slowly, and the end-position should be held still. None of the stretches should cause you any pain or discomfort.

Back stretch (Figure 1)

- Lying on your back, bring your knees up towards your chest.
- Draw your knees into your chest, using your arms to help.
- You should feel a stretch in your lower back.
- Hold for a count of _____ .
- Repeat _____ times.

Quadriceps stretch (Figure 2)

- Lie on your tummy on the bed.
- Press your hips firmly into the bed and bring your foot up towards your buttocks. Take hold of the foot with your hand and ease the foot closer to your buttocks.
- You should feel a stretch in the front of your thigh.
- Hold for a count of _____ .
- Repeat _____ times.
- Repeat with the other leg.

Figure 1

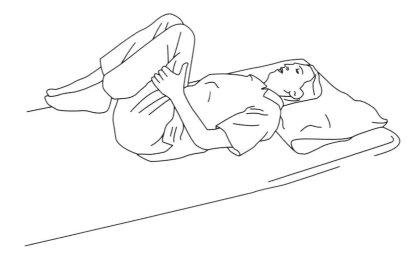

Figure 2

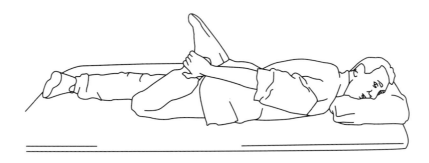

Hip flexor stretch (prone) (Figure 3)

- Lie on your tummy on the bed.
- Keeping your hips flat down onto the bed, lift your shoulders up and rest on your elbows.
- You should feel a stretch in the front of your hips.
- Hold for a count of _____ .
- Repeat _____ times.
- If leaning on your elbows is difficult, you can just lie flat on your tummy and try and flatten your hips onto the bed.

Hip flexor stretch (supine) (Figure 4)

- If lying on your tummy is difficult, you can also stretch your hip muscles by sitting on the edge of the bed and lying back.
- You may need to rest your feet on a book if the bed is high, so your feet are resting flat.
- You should feel a stretch in the front of your hips and thighs.
- Try not to let your lower back arch.
- Hold for a count of _____ .
- Repeat _____ times.

Figure 3

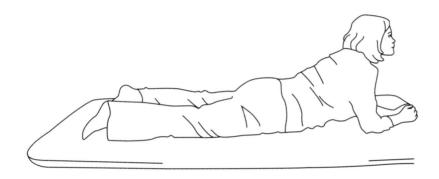

Figure 4

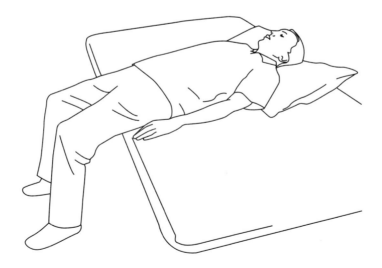

Hip adductor stretch (Figure 5)

- In a sitting position, bend your hips and knees up and place the soles of your feet together (you can sit cross-legged if this is easier).
- Lean gently onto your thighs with your elbows and push down towards the floor.
- You should feel a stretch on your inner thighs.
- Hold for a count of _____ .
- Repeat _____ times.

Hamstring stretch (Figure 6)

- Sit near the edge of the bed, with one leg on the bed and the other one over the side with the foot flat on the floor.
- Keeping the back of your knee flat to the bed, lean forwards, reaching your hands towards your ankle.
- You will feel a stretch in the back of your thigh.
- Hold for a count of _____ .
- Repeat _____ times.
- Then perform this same movement on the opposite side.

Figure 5

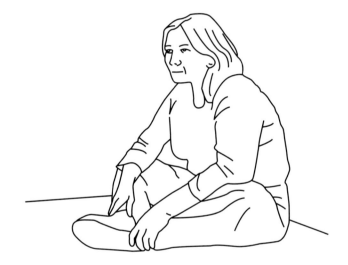

Figure 6

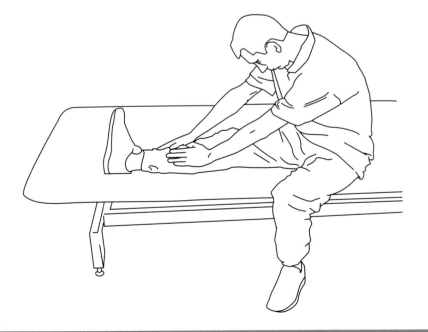

Calf stretch (gastrocnemius muscle) (Figure 7)

- Stand with one foot in front of the other, resting your hands on a table or wall for balance.
- Keeping the back leg *straight*, slowly lean towards the wall, allowing the front knee to bend.
- A comfortable stretch should be felt in the calf of the rear leg.
- Hold for a count of _____ .
- Repeat _____ times.
- Then perform this same movement on the opposite side.

Calf stretch (soleus muscle) (Figure 8)

- Stand with one foot in front of the other, resting your hands on a wall or table for balance.
- Keeping the back leg *slightly bent*, slowly lean towards the wall, allowing your front knee to bend.
- A comfortable stretch should be felt in the lower part of the calf of the rear leg.
- Hold for a count of _____ .
- Repeat _____ times.
- Then perform this same movement on the opposite side.

Figure 7

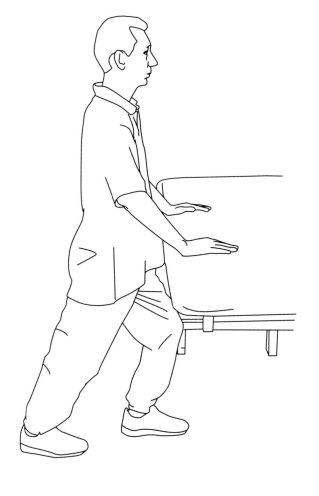

Figure 8

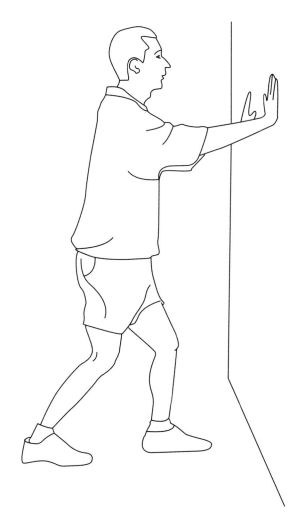

Wrist and finger stretch (Figure 9)

- Sit on the edge of the bed or on a firm chair.
- Place your hand so that your fingers are facing backwards.
- Keep your elbow straight and lean your weight down through your arm.
- You should feel a stretch in your forearm.
- Hold for a count of _____ .
- Repeat _____ times.
- Repeat, if needed, on the opposite side.

Assisted calf stretch (Figure 10)

- Rest the person's heel in the palm of your hand and your forearm along the sole of their foot. Place your other hand further up the leg, holding just below the knee.
- Slowly move the foot upward towards the body at the same time as pulling the heel down.
- The person should feel a stretch in the back of their calf.
- Hold for a count of _____ .
- Repeat _____ times.
- Repeat on the other leg.

Figure 9

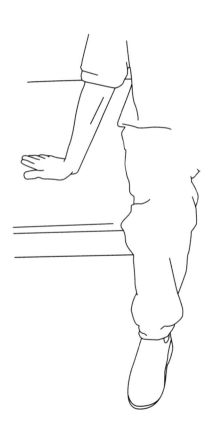

Figure 10

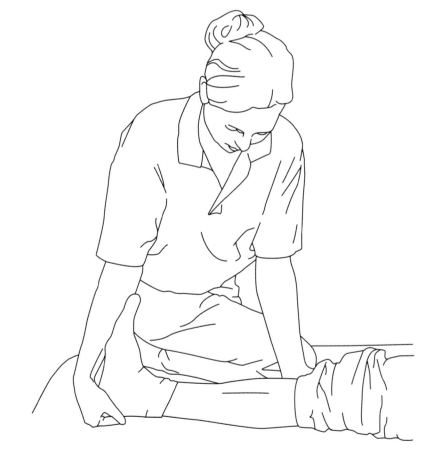

Assisted back stretch (Figure 11)

- Start with the person lying flat on their back.
- Holding below the knee joints, slowly bend their knees and hips up towards their chest.
- The person should feel a stretch in their lower back.
- Hold for a count of_____ .
- Repeat _____ times.

Assisted hip adductor stretch (Figure 12)

- Start with the person positioned on their back, with their knees bent and feet flat on the bed.
- With your hands placed on their inner thighs above the knees, slowly move the knees apart.
- The person should feel a stretch in their inner thighs.
- Hold for a count of _____ .
- Repeat _____ times.

Figure 11

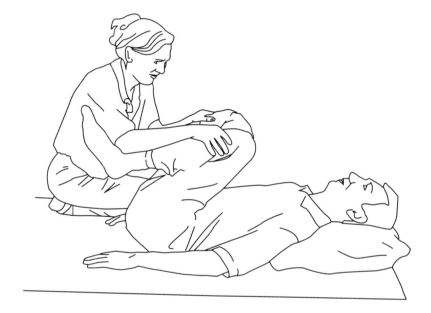

Figure 12

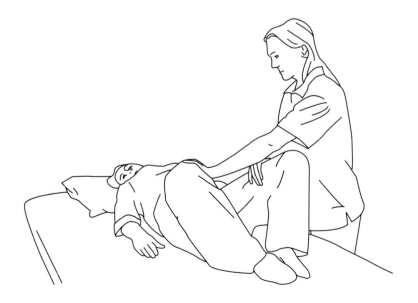

Hamstring stretch (Figure 13)

- Start with the person positioned lying on their back.
- Raise one leg up, keeping the knee bent.
- Slowly try to straighten the knee, keeping the thigh still.
- The person should feel a stretch in the back of their thigh.
- Hold for a count of _____ .
- Repeat _____ times.
- Repeat with the opposite leg.

What to do if:

1. You are getting clonus while trying to stretch (Figure 14)

- Try to keep your weight on the affected leg.
- If standing, transfer your weight onto the leg and push down through the heel.
- If sitting, bend the knee and press down onto your thigh, pushing the heel onto the floor.

2. You get spasms while trying to stretch

- Try to get into a comfortable position before you start, and stretch slowly.
- If you get a spasm, stop the movement, let it pass, and then continue.
- Changing the time of day you carry out the stretches or having help from another person may reduce the number of spasms you experience.
- If you take medication to help with muscle spasms or stiffness, try to take it at least 20 minutes before starting your stretches.

3. Fatigue makes exercise difficult

- Exercise at times of the day when you feel less tired, for example in the morning or after having a rest.
- If fatigue is a significant problem for you, incorporate regular rests into your stretching programme.

Figure 13

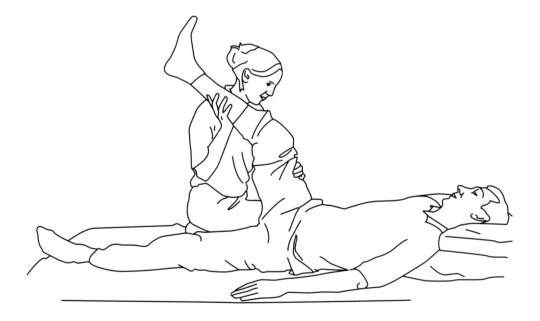

Figure 14

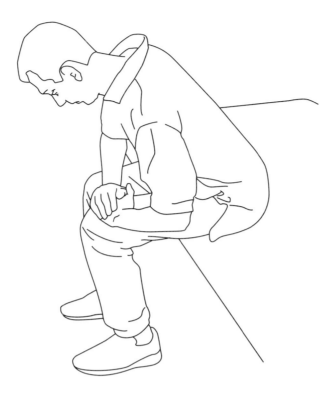

4. It is difficult to fit exercise into the day

- Incorporate stretches where possible into your daily activities, such as when you are watching the television or listening to the radio.

5. You get pain while carrying out one of the stretches

- Stop doing the specific stretch that causes the pain, and seek advice from your physiotherapist or doctor.

6. You need help to carry out these stretches

- Discuss this with your physiotherapist when selecting the stretches you need to do. It is often possible for the physiotherapist to demonstrate the stretches to another person such as a family member or carer.

If you are unsure about carrying out any of these stretches please contact your physiotherapist or doctor for advice. Their contact details are listed below:

_____

_____

_____

_____

_____

_____

Appendix 5

How botulinum toxin may help your limb spasticity

What is botulinum toxin?

Botulinum toxin is a chemical that is normally produced by a naturally occurring bacterium. When it is injected into muscles, it temporarily weakens them. The toxin works by blocking the communication between the nerves and muscles. As a result of the injection, the muscles become weaker and less stiff, and this can help in the management of the condition.

Why give injections?

The doctors and therapists who are assessing you have identified that there is a problem with excessive muscle activity that is occurring as a result of damage to the brain or spinal cord from a stroke or a condition such as multiple sclerosis. These problems may include pain, stiffness and difficulty moving the limb, which in turn may lead to difficulties with day-to-day activities such as washing and dressing. Other difficulties may include participating in a therapy stretching programme to maintain good muscle length, which may include putting on and off splints or other orthotic devices. The toxin is injected to weaken a particular muscle that is causing the problem so that the muscle can be stretched and moved more easily.

How are the injections given?

The injections are given in the clinic. The muscles to be injected are identified by physical examination, and then a special needle is inserted into the muscle. Sometimes the needle is connected to an EMG (electromyography) machine: this registers the electrical activity of the muscle and helps to guide the correct placement of the injection. By physical examination and EMG, we can help ensure that the toxin only goes into the muscles that we want to become less stiff. Several muscles may need to be injected.

Botulinum toxin injections are no more painful than any other common injections such as tetanus vaccinations. The number of injections given depends on the number of muscles that are overactive.

How long will it take?

It will take about 30 minutes to complete the assessment and injection.

What happens after the injection?

Botulinum toxin takes 1–3 days to begin to work, and usually reaches its peak around 1–3 weeks later. Some muscles and some people respond faster than others. The muscles injected should become less stiff. The reduction in stiffness depends on how tight the muscles were before the injection, how sensitive you are to the toxin and how much toxin is injected. The effect of the toxin can wear off after a period of time.

A specific exercise programme involving either stretches or active exercises of the limb injected will help to maximise the effect of the injection. The team will arrange for you to be assessed by a physiotherapist or occupational therapist after the injections so that the programme can be tailored to your individual needs.

What are the side-effects?

Reported side-effects include a skin rash, flu-like illness and tiredness, but they tend to be mild and short-lived. They are uncommon and tend not to require any treatment. Another rare complication can be difficulty swallowing, but this tends to be associated with injections into neck muscles, which we rarely do in the spasticity clinic.

If you are at all concerned about side-effects following the injection, please contact your GP.

Goal of treatment

It is important to set a goal for the botulinum toxin injections so that you have an aim to work towards and for evaluation of the effectiveness of the treatment.

Goal

_____

_____

_____

_____

_____

Date: _____

Therapy follow-up arrangements

_____

_____

_____

Appendix 6

How intrathecal baclofen therapy may help to manage your spasticity

What is spasticity?

Spasticity can be described as involuntary muscle stiffness. It is a common symptom of neurological disease, and can range from mild to severe and change over time, often from day to day or hour to hour. Other associated features can include spasms, pain, weakness and clonus. Spasticity is not always detrimental, as some people use the stiffness in their muscles to help them stand, transfer or walk. However, prolonged spasticity may result in shortening of the muscle, which further increases the stiffness, limits the range of movement of the limb and is not always responsive to drug treatments.

Why does spasticity occur?

Nerve pathways connecting the brain, spinal cord and muscles work together to coordinate movements of the body. Disruption of these pathways, particularly in the spinal cord, can lead to spasticity and spasms.

How is spasticity managed?

Most people with mild to moderate spasticity can control their symptoms with exercises (including standing and stretches), physiotherapy, prevention of aggravating symptoms and oral anti-spasticity drugs.

However, despite treatment and prevention of trigger factors, spasticity can become severe and difficult to manage, affecting all aspects of daily life. Intrathecal baclofen may be considered at this stage.

Aggravating factors

- Urinary retention or infections
- Bowel impaction, constipation
- Red or broken skin areas
- Poor positions in lying or sitting
- Tight-fitting clothes or splints
- Pain
- Infections
- Low mood

What is baclofen?

Baclofen is an anti-spasticity drug used to help control muscle stiffness and spasms. It acts by reducing the transfer of signals to and from specific nerve receptors found in the spinal cord and brain; this dampens down the effects of spasticity and its associated symptoms. It is usually taken orally as a tablet.

Does oral anti-spasticity medication work for everyone?

No – some people find that oral doses of anti-spasticity medication can help relieve their spasticity a little, but not totally, while others find the side-effects unacceptable. Common side-effects from oral baclofen can include weakness, drowsiness, fatigue and dizziness.

Why can baclofen sometimes fail when taken orally as a tablet?

The brain has a protective mechanism known as the blood–brain barrier, which prevents unwanted substances and sometimes drugs entering into the nervous system. When taken orally, it is difficult for baclofen to pass through the blood–brain barrier. This can result in too much baclofen in the bloodstream, causing side-effects (weakness, drowsiness and dizziness), and too little in the spinal cord to relieve spasticity.

What is 'intrathecal'?

'Intrathecal' refers to a space surrounding the spinal cord; this space is filled with cerebrospinal fluid (CSF). The CSF circulates around the brain and spinal cord, acting as a shock absorber to protect these delicate structures.

Why should baclofen work when administered intrathecally?

Concentrations of the nerve receptors sensitive to baclofen are found in the spinal cord. Giving baclofen intrathecally allows it to be delivered directly to the specific receptors. As the drug is being delivered directly onto the receptor sites, only small doses need to be used (about 100th of the oral dose). This can mean that the side-effects such as drowsiness experienced with oral doses can be less of a problem.

Does baclofen work for everyone intrathecally?

No – some people do not respond to baclofen given intrathecally. A trial of the drug is necessary to see if a person responds to it.

Preparing for the trial

At the National Hospital for Neurology and Neurosurgery (NHNN), the trial stage begins with admission to a neurology or rehabilitation ward.

Day 1 or 2

- The medical and nursing teams will spend some time with you asking about your symptoms and finding out the best way to support your care needs while in hospital.

- In the spasticity assessment clinic, education about the trial and written information would have been provided; the clinical nurse specialist for spasticity management (CNS) will recap on the trial procedure, provide further copies of the written information if needed and answer any further queries you may have.

- The CNS and a physiotherapist (PT) who specialises in managing spasticity will jointly assess your spasticity and spasms: this will involve moving and stretching your limbs. If you have pain, they will only move you within the range that is tolerable. A baseline set of measures will be recorded (including the frequency of your spasms, how your limbs feel when stretched and how comfortable you feel). Together, you will decide on a main goal of treatment. These aims and measures are valuable, as after each trial you and the team can evaluate whether the intrathecal baclofen improves your spasticity. This can help you and the team decide if it would be an effective treatment for you in the long-term.

What happens in the trial?

- The trial injection allows relatively large amounts of baclofen to enter your CSF; it is at this stage that the nurses and doctors will be particularly vigilant in monitoring your condition for signs of having too much baclofen (see the box for a list of potential side-effects). The trial dose is not a permanent treatment: it will reach maximum effect 4–6 hours after injection and will then start to wear off. So, if you do experience side-effects, they will reduce as the drug level in your body reduces. At worse your breathing could be affected and you may require support in an intensive care unit overnight: this enables you to be closely monitored until the drug wears off completely and your breathing is no longer affected.

The three most common side-effects of baclofen overdose

- Drowsiness
- Weakness of legs
- Dizziness/light-headedness

Other side-effects

Seizures
Nausea/vomiting
Low or high blood pressure
Constipation
Slurred speech
Weakness in arms
Difficulty breathing
Headache
Numbness/itching/tingling
Blurred vision
Low tone
Lethargy

Day 2 or 3

- You will be given an opportunity to discuss the trial procedure and your goal for the treatment with the consultant neurologist or a member of the senior medical team. You, together with the whole multidisciplinary team, will decide whether to continue with the trial.
- A doctor will ask you to sign a consent form to agree to the trial procedure.
- If you proceed with the trial, a doctor will administer a dose of 25 micrograms (µg) of intrathecal baclofen via a lumbar puncture into your intrathecal space; the trial is carried out on the ward. The first dose will be given before 12:00 noon. This enables accurate evaluation of the response by you and the team 4 hours later, when it reaches maximum effect.
- Following the injection, you will be requested to remain on bed rest for 1–2 hours. During this time, the nursing staff will check regularly to see how you feel and will perform close observations of the oxygen levels in your blood (using a small monitor attached to one of your fingers) and your pulse, blood pressure, breathing and limb power. They will also monitor for signs of drowsiness or other side-effects.

- When the dose peaks, the CNS and PT will measure your response at this time and assess with you whether your goal could be achieved.
- If you do not respond, the procedure can be repeated over the next 2–3 days by gradually increasing the bolus dose to 50, 75 and 100 µg.

How many trials will I need?

At least two trials will be done on separate days. As you know, spasticity and spasms can vary from day to day, so it is important that we see an effect on two separate occasions.

Non-responsive – what next?

The maximum dose of baclofen given at the trial stage is 100 µg. If you do not respond to a dose of 100 µg or less, this therapy is unsuitable. In this case, your consultant neurologist will advise on alternative treatments.

Responsive – what next?

If you respond to baclofen, the CNS will provide education and information on having an internal pump implanted that could provide you with long-term treatment. The consultant neurologist will be available to discuss all options. If, following discussion and time to absorb all the information, you decide to have the pump implanted, this will be arranged by the CNS. The implantation date will depend on the availability of key team members, and may result in you going home for a short while with a follow-up date for re-admission.

What does a pump system consist of?

The pump system consists of a reservoir and catheter (Figure 1). The reservoir stores the intrathecal baclofen and the catheter connects the reservoir to the CSF in the intrathecal space around the spinal cord (Figure 2). The reservoir is a round metal disk about 8.5 cm (3.5 inches) in diameter and 2 cm (0.75 inch) in depth. It weighs about 165 g (6 ounces). Two pump sizes are available: one has a 20 ml and the other a 40 ml reservoir. The latter pump is slightly bigger – we regularly use the 20 ml pump.

How is the pump implanted?

The pump is implanted under general anaesthetic by a neurosurgeon in theatre. The pump is placed under the skin in the abdomen, and a catheter connects it to the intrathecal space around the spinal cord so that the complete system remains hidden under the skin (Figure 2). The procedure, including being anaesthetised, the operation and time in the recovery room, can take approximately 2–4 hours. The pump is filled with baclofen in theatre and programmed with a daily dose in the recovery room. Once you are fully recovered from the anaesthetic, you will return to the ward.

Programming the pump

The reservoir has a microchip inside it, which allows the amount of drug to be programmed using a specific computer called a telemeter (Figure 3). To programme the pump, the telemeter is placed lightly on the skin over the pump.

Alarms

The pump has an alarm, which will sound if there is a problem. You will be told exactly what to do if this should ever happen.

Does the pump work right away?

Yes – the pump will be programmed to deliver the intrathecal baclofen at the prescribed rate as soon as you are awake following the surgery.

Figure 1

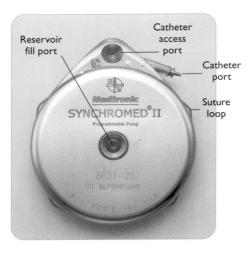

Pump (SynchroMed II, Medtronic, 2004)

Figure 3

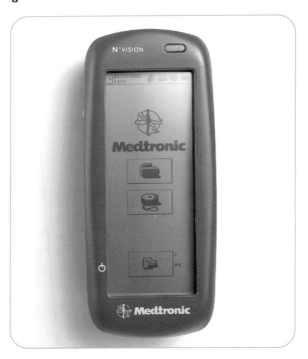

Telemeter to programme the pump

Figure 2

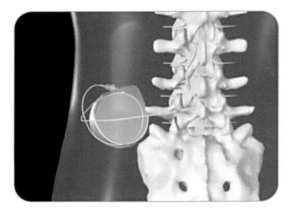

Positioning of pump and catheter

Will the response be the same as the trial?

No – during the trial, you will have received a relatively large, one-off dose of baclofen to assess whether you respond to it. To administer it safely and effectively over time, much smaller amounts are required, and are delivered continuously at an hourly rate. It may therefore be a few days before you feel the benefit of the therapy.

Once the pump is in place, the next step is to find the dose most suited to you as an individual. The aim is to find the dose that decreases spasticity enough to achieve the set goals without causing unwanted side-effects. This process takes time, and so it is important to appreciate that it may take 3–6 months or longer to find the dose suitable for you as an individual. It is therefore unlikely that your optimum dose will be achieved before you leave hospital.

The outpatient process of assessing your spasticity, titrating the dose and refilling your pump occurs in a specific clinic in the outpatients department. This is known as the 'pump' clinic.

How long will I be in hospital?

The average length of stay in hospital for both a trial and pump implantation is 10–14 days.

What are my responsibilities?

Before discharge from hospital, you will have received extensive education regarding pump management from the CNS. You will also receive written information to take home with you.

It is your responsibility to:

- Contact the hospital if you feel there is a problem with the pump.
- Know the signs of overdose and underdose.
- Know the correct contact procedure for non-urgent problems.
- Know the emergency contact procedure.
- Attend the outpatients department as scheduled for refills and changes of prescription.

How is the level of baclofen in my reservoir monitored?

The CNS will monitor the dates that your pump will require refilling and will liaise with you about when you need to attend an outpatient clinic. This can vary between 1 and 6 months. In the clinic, the CNS and a doctor will review your current dose and how well your spasticity is being managed, and your pump reservoir will be refilled. You will need to attend the clinic to have regular refills.

Refills involve placing a needle through the skin into the pump's refill port and reservoir; this procedure may be uncomfortable, but is not usually painful (Figure 4). The old baclofen is withdrawn and fresh baclofen is inserted. The pump is then programmed to deliver the prescribed drug dose.

Common questions

In the past, people considering intrathecal baclofen have asked us the following questions, which we have included here for your information.

Oral doses of anti-spasticity drugs (e.g. baclofen and tizanidine) – Do I keep taking them?

Yes – it is important that your oral anti-spasticity doses are slowly reduced under the guidance of your medical team while in hospital and when followed-up in the pump refill clinic.

Will the pump cure my underlying condition?

No – it is important to appreciate that the pump is useful only in managing the symptoms of spasticity and spasms. It will not cure your neurological condition or influence its course.

Will the pump be visible?

Pumps are usually not visible under clothes. However, if you are very slim and wear tight clothing, an outline of the pump may be seen. Before implantation of the pump, you will be given an opportunity by the CNS to wear a prototype pump taped to your skin. This will help you to decide the best position for the pump, taking into consideration the position of your

Figure 4

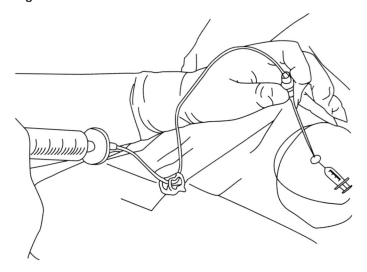

Illustration of a pump being refilled

waistbands and belts and comfort when sitting and lying and during sexual intercourse.

Can I wash and shower with a pump?

Yes – it is okay to wash and shower with a pump in place. Initially, following the surgery, you will have stitches or clips at the wound. These must be kept dry until the wound is healed: usually 7–10 days. The nursing staff will advise you on how to keep the wound dry when washing during this period.

Is it okay to have sex with a pump in place?

Yes – some people have expressed concern that the pump may be displaced or damaged during sexual intercourse. The pump is placed in a deep pocket in the abdomen, so it is well protected.

Will I be able to travel abroad with a pump?

Yes – it may be possible for the CNS to liaise with the pump manufacturer (Medtronic), to help identify contact names and telephone numbers in case of an emergency when travelling abroad. You must check before travelling abroad that you have enough baclofen in the pump to cover your time away. Before discharge, the CNS will give you an identification card that will detail the type of pump and drug you have – it is advisable to carry this with you at all times

in case of emergency. Note that your pump may set off metal detectors at airports, so present your identification card to the security personnel.

How long does the pump last?

The battery that powers the pump lasts approximately 5–7 years.

A planned admission will be arranged for replacement of the pump following discussion with your neurologist. The replacement involves removing the pump from the abdomen and attaching a new pump to the existing catheter; this is usually performed under general anaesthetic to facilitate proper positioning.

Is it possible to be cremated with a pump?

Some people have expressed concern about this issue. If you plan to be cremated, please note that the pump needs to be removed by the funeral directors prior to the cremation. The removal of medical devices is regular practice for undertakers, so they will be used to doing this.

Can I take other medications?

You may need to take other medications when you have an implanted pump. Your GP will be aware of any contraindications, and can always seek advice from your neurologist as necessary.

Will the pump interfere with my daily activities?

The presence of the pump should not curtail your lifestyle. Overall, you may find that the pump increases your ability to participate in daily activities. For many people, a reduction in spasm leads to an improved quality of life.

What support is available when I am at home?

- Your GP will receive information on intrathecal baclofen and the contact procedures.
- If other healthcare members are involved in your daily life, copies of information packs will be made available as necessary.

- The CNS is available to offer advice and education to your community and social care team as needed.
- The CNS is available Monday to Friday during office hours. Out-of-hours advice is available through the nurse in charge on the ward.

If your questions have not been answered in this leaflet or if you wish to discuss things further, please contact:

_____

_____

_____

Appendix 7

Medical procedure for intrathecal baclofen trial injection

1. Obtain the individual's consent for at least two trials (two positive results are required before an implant can be considered).
2. Plan to complete the procedure before 12:00 noon.
3. Assemble equipment for a lumbar puncture plus an antibacterial filter, 5 ml syringe, intrathecal baclofen (normally in solution of 50 µg/ml) and 5 ml of sterile normal saline.
4. Dilute the required dose of intrathecal baclofen with normal saline to make a solution of 5 ml.
5. Connect the filter to the 5 ml syringe and prime with the baclofen solution. Place the prepared syringe back onto the sterile field.
6. Perform a lumbar puncture using a sterile procedure.
7. Connect to the spinal needle and inject the solution over 2–3 minutes.
8. Ask the ward nurses to monitor as per protocol in the care plan, and feedback immediately if any adverse events occur.
9. Ask the person to gradually sit up over the next 1–2 hours. They can get out of bed to use the toilet. However, they will need strict supervision when getting out, as they may experience significant tone changes, which alters the way they transfer and mobilise.
10. If side-effects are experienced with the initial dose, discuss with the spasticity management team before proceeding to the second dose.
11. A positive response needs to have an effect that lasts for at least 6 hours post the peak time.

Appendix 8

Nursing care plans for intrathecal baclofen therapy

INTRATHECAL BACLOFEN TRIAL CARE PLAN		Name: Hospital No.:
Problem 1	**Expected outcome**	**Nursing intervention**
Person with spasticity (PWS) requires information and education to make an informed decision about proceeding with the trial of intrathecal baclofen (ITB) therapy Baclofen acts by binding to γ-aminobutyric acid (GABA) receptors. It has a presynaptic inhibitory effect on the release of excitatory neurotransmitters[1] and postsynaptically it decreases the firing of motor neurones.[2] This results in inhibition of mono- and polysynaptic spinal reflexes,[3] with associated reductions in spasm, clonus and pain. Delivering baclofen intrathecally accentuates its anti-spasticity effect while minimising the troublesome systemic side-effects associated with oral intake	PWS makes an informed decision	• Liaise with spasticity clinical nurse specialist (CNS) • CNS to educate and inform person of the process, with a member of ward nursing staff present • Ward nurses to reinforce information as necessary and continue teaching Education/information should include: **A description of procedure:** A bolus dose of baclofen is inserted into the intrathecal space via a spinal needle **The care required after injection:** The drug peaks 4 hours after injection. This is a critical time for the nurse and PWS to assess the effect of the drug and to monitor for side-effects. See multidisciplinary protocol and Problem 2

Problem 2	Expected outcome	Nursing intervention
(a) A spasticity assessment and baseline measures need to be recorded pre intrathecal trial injection	Accurate record of spasticity and spasms to ascertain efficacy of treatment	• CNS and physiotherapist (PT) will complete an assessment and measures pre and post injections • Nurses to give feedback on how spasticity affects nursing care
(b) Main problem and goal of treatment need to be established[4]	Agreed goal: _____ _____ _____	• Medical team, CNS and PT will discuss and agree goal with PWS
(c) Changes in level of spasticity throughout admission may affect PWS's ability to carry out activities or to be cared for	Accurate identification of any changes in function	• Identify any changes in level of function and assist with care as required to promote safety • Liaise with spasticity management team
(d) PWS is at risk of overdose or adverse reaction to ITB[5]	PWS aware of associated side-effects pre trial and know what to report	• Nurses to familiarise themselves with level of spasticity/stiffness felt in the PWS's limbs and the frequency and intensity of spasms prior to treatment to enable assessment of changes post injection • Record neurological observations, blood pressure (BP), pulse, respiration (resp.) rate and oxygen saturations pre treatment
(e) The trial attempts to assess if ITB will improve current spasticity management of PWS. Therefore the current spasticity management strategies need to continue	PWS will continue their regular spasticity management strategies	• Continue with normal spasticity management, i.e. oral drug regime, stretching programme, and effective management of bladder and bowels • **The PWS will continue to take normal oral drugs unless indicated by the medical team throughout the trial period. If side-effects occur, contact medical team**
(f) Anti-emboli stockings are rarely required for people having ITB therapy	To prevent skin breakdown	• Often in people with severe spasticity and spasms, anti-emboli stockings are difficult to apply and keep in a position that will promote skin integrity. Passive limb exercises are the preferred method of preventing deep-vein thrombosis (DVT)
Problem 3	**Expected outcome**	**Nursing intervention**
(a) ITB to be administered by medical team	Drug will peak 4–6 hours following the dose, and will then gradually wear off	Doctors to inject drug before 12:00 noon, ensuring peak time occurs when most of team is on duty **Date of trial 1:** _____ Time of injection: _____ Time of peak: _____ **Date of trial 2:** _____ Time of injection: _____ Time of peak: _____

(b) Bolus injections of ITB permit a large amount of the drug to enter the cerebrospinal fluid (CSF). Side-effects are most likely to occur at this time[6]	Signs of overdose are recognised early and prompt action is taken	**Post-injection observations:** • Pulse, BP, resp. rate and oxygen saturations: **½-hourly for 2 hours** **1-hourly for 4 hours** **2-hourly for 2 hours** **4-hourly unless patient's condition dictates otherwise** • Record pulse oximetry for at least 4 hours post injection • Record neurological observations 1-hourly for 6 hours Monitor the patient and encourage them to report any signs of overdose: • **Drowsiness** • **Weakness in limbs** • **Dizziness/light-headedness** • **Diplopia** • **Nausea/vomiting** • **Depressed respiration**
(c) IV physostigmine can help to reverse central side-effects.[7] It should only be given by a doctor after consultation with an anaesthetist, as it has been reported to cause cardiac arrhythmias[8]	Emergency treatment is available	• Ensure that IV physostigmine is available on the ward and not expired (it has a short shelf-life) • Ensure access to ventilatory support/resuscitation trolley **Report any significant changes to nurse-in-charge/doctors promptly**
Problem 4	**Expected outcome**	**Nursing intervention**
PWS may develop a headache as a result of the intrathecal injection causing a CSF leak	• PWS will report symptoms of headache • PWS will report any headache pain being under control	• Encourage at least 2 litres of fluid intake over 24 hours • Encourage PWS to gradually sit up post procedure • PWS can get up to go to the toilet, but will need supervision or assistance when transferring and mobilising, as their tone could have changed • If headache starts, encourage PWS to lie flat and then inform the medical team • Offer analgesia as prescribed, and monitor its effectiveness • Inform doctors if analgesia is ineffective • If PWS is unable to tolerate oral fluids, depending on the severity of the headache, it may be necessary to commence IV fluids

Problem 5	Expected outcome	Nursing intervention
PWS together with team need to decide whether to go ahead with a pump implant	PWS is able to make an informed decision	PWS, spasticity team and ward nurses discuss outcome of trials, and whether: • Agreed goal would be achieved • PWS is willing to take on responsibility for the pump • PWS wishes to proceed to implant Depending on outcome the CNS will arrange follow up or proceed to implant

INTRATHECAL BACLOFEN PUM INSERTION CARE PLAN		Name: Hospital No.:
Problem I	**Expected outcome**	**Nursing intervention**
(a) Person with spasticity (PWS) needs to be aware of the implications of treatment with intrathecal baclofen (ITB) and their responsibilities in the management of a pump implant[9]	They are able to discuss the implant process as well as their responsibilities and whom to contact in an emergency situation	Spasticity clinical nurse specialist (CNS) to discuss with PWS: • Procedure for pump implant • Follow-up refills, and titration of dose • Potential side-effects • How the alarms function • Emergency contact procedure
(b) Main problem and goal of intervention need to be identified and agreed between team members and PWS[4]	Agreed goal: _____ _____ _____	• Nurses and PWS monitor achievement of goal and feedback to team
(c) PWS needs to explore optimum site for the pump to be implanted: either the right or left side of their abdomen	For PWS to state they are happy with proposed site of implant	• Nurses to assist PWS to tape a prototype pump to their abdomen and to try different sitting and lying positions. Consider position of waistbands in the different positions • Nurses liaise with CNS, to mark the skin for preferred site for implant • Ensure choice recorded on pre-operative sheet

Problem 2	Expected outcome	Nursing intervention
(a) PWS needs to be safely prepared for theatre	They state they feel informed and ready for theatre	• CNS to discuss procedure for implant with PWS • PWS will be seen by an anaesthetist and surgical team pre-operatively, who will obtain consent • For ward nurses to follow pre-operative procedure as per hospital policy
(b) Anti-emboli stockings are rarely required for people having ITB therapy	To prevent skin breakdown	• Often in people with severe spasticity and spasms, anti-emboli stockings are difficult to apply and keep in a position that will promote skin integrity. Passive limb exercises are the preferred method of preventing deep-vein thrombosis (DVT)
Problem 3	**Expected outcome**	**Nursing intervention**
(a) PWS needs to recover safely from anaesthetic	PWS is monitored and a safe recovery is promoted at all times	• PWS will go to recovery and will remain there until at least 30 minutes after the catheter has been primed and the ITB dose commenced
(b) Potential for baclofen overdosage/underdosage[5,6]	Signs of overdose/underdose will be reported and treated promptly	• On return to ward, neurological and general observations need to be completed: **½-hourly for 2 hours** **1-hourly for 4 hours** **2-hourly for 2 hours** **4-hourly unless their condition dictates otherwise** Monitor patient and encourage them to report any **signs of overdose:** • **Drowsiness** • **Weakness in limbs** • **Dizziness/light-headedness** • **Diplopia** • **Nausea/vomiting** • **Depressed respiration**
(c) IV physostigmine can help to reverse central side-effects.[7] It should only be given by a doctor and after consultation with an anaesthetist, as it has been reported to cause cardiac arrhythmias[8]	Signs of overdose are identified early and appropriate treatment is available	Report any signs of overdose to CNS and medical team. If an emergency, contact the on-call anaesthetist. Ensure access to: • IV physostigmine on the ward (ensure that it has not expired – it has a short shelf-life) • Pump programmer • Refill kit • Resuscitation trolley

Problem 4	Expected outcome	Nursing intervention
Risk of infection/haematoma at wound sites[4]	Any signs of infection/meningitis/haematoma will be detected and treatment commenced promptly	Observe lumbar and abdomen wound sites for signs of: • Redness • Swelling • Tenderness 4-hourly temperatures until discharge **Clip removal** Abdomen 7 days Date: _____ Lumbar 10 days Date: _____ If patient is to be discharged before date of clip removal, organise for district nurse to remove clips and send patient home with clip remover
Problem 5	**Expected outcome**	**Nursing intervention**
Changes in level of spasticity throughout the admission may affect PWS's ability to carry out activities or to be cared for	Changes in function are detected early and appropriate action taken	• Identify any changes in level of function, and assist with care as required to promote safety • Liaise with spasticity and community teams
Problem 6	**Expected outcome**	**Nursing intervention**
(a) PWS needs to feel prepared to go home with new implant in situ[9]	PWS (or nominated carer) knows about the treatment and its implications	• CNS to give verbal and written information on pump, side-effects, emergency contact procedure and alarm systems • Nurses to ensure that PWS and/or carer are able to describe side-effects and what action they would take in an emergency • CNS to give PWS pump identification card • CNS to demonstrate alarm system to PWS and family • CNS to arrange follow-up in outpatient spasticity review and refill clinic • Nurses to ensure PWS and carer are aware of review date
(b) Community team need to be aware of discharge and that an intrathecal pump has been implanted	Community team state they have received enough information	• Medical team to contact GP • Nurses to contact district nurse • Nurses to ensure ward clerk sends information pack to GP and community teams at least 2 days before discharge

INTRATHECAL BACLOFEN REPLACEMENT PUMP INSERTION CARE PLAN		Name: Hospital No.:
Problem I	**Expected outcome**	**Nursing intervention**
(a) Person with spasticity (PWS) needs to consider implications for pump replacement and confirm they wish to proceed	PWS is able to discuss their responsibilities and state how they would access emergency help	Spasticity clinical nurse specialist (CNS) to discuss: • Procedure for pump replacement • Potential of a period of increase in spasticity following the implant • Confirm whether PWS wishes to proceed CNS will recap on: • Follow-up process and titration of dose • Potential side-effects • How alarms function • Emergency contact procedure
(b) PWS to confirm whether they want the pump re-implanted in the same position or whether they wish to change it (NB: Changing the side of the pump implant would necessitate a catheter change as well)	PWS states they are happy with the proposed site of implant	• CNS and ward nurses to confirm with PWS their preferred site for implant – taking into consideration any problems they may have had with the current position • Ensure choice recorded on pre-operative sheet
(c) Need to assess PWS's baseline spasticity. The main problem and goal of intervention need to be identified and agreed between team members and PWS[4]	To ensure that their spasticity is effectively managed post-operatively Agreed goal: _____ _____	• CNS and physiotherapist (PT) to assess spasticity pre and post treatment • Nurses to monitor achievement of goal and feedback to team
Problem 2	**Expected outcome**	**Nursing intervention**
(a) PWS needs to be safely prepared for theatre	PWS states they feel informed and ready for theatre	CNS to discuss procedure for implant with PWS, aided by ward nurses: • They will be reviewed by the spasticity team, an anaesthetist and neurosurgical team pre-operatively; the latter will obtain consent • Nurses to follow pre-operative procedure as per hospital policy
(b) Anti-emboli stockings are rarely required for people having ITB therapy	To prevent skin breakdown	• Often in people with severe spasticity and spasms, anti-emboli stockings are difficult to apply and keep in a position that will promote skin integrity. Passive limb exercises are the preferred method of preventing deep-vein thrombosis (DVT)

Problem 3	Expected outcome	Nursing intervention
(a) PWS needs to recover safely from anaesthetic	PWS is monitored and a safe recovery is promoted at all times	• PWS will go to recovery and will remain there for at least 30 minutes after the ITB dose has commenced • On return to ward, neurological and general observations need to be completed: **½-hourly for 2 hours** **1-hourly for 4 hours** **2-hourly for 2 hours** **4-hourly unless otherwise required**
(b) Potential for baclofen overdosage/underdosage[5,6]	Signs of overdose/underdose will be reported and treated promptly	If the person is underdosed, they will experience spasms/increased spasticity (stiffness) of their lower limbs. Report this to CNS and medical team Monitor PWS and encourage them to report any **signs of overdose**: • **Drowsiness** • **Weakness in limbs** • **Dizziness/light-headedness** • **Diplopia** • **Nausea/vomiting** • **Depressed respiration**
(c) IV physostigmine can help to reverse central side-effects.[7] It should only be given by a doctor and after consultation with an anaesthetist, as it has been reported to cause cardiac arrhythmias[8]	Ensure IV physostigmine is available if needed	Report any signs of overdose to CNS and medical team. If an emergency, contact the on-call anaesthetist Ensure access to • IV physostigmine on the ward (ensure it has not expired – it has a short shelf-life) • Pump programmer • Refill kit • Resuscitation trolley
(d) Some PWS experience a period of increased spasticity following the replacement if some ITB was lost when the new pump was connected to the catheter	PWS and ward nurses to be aware if increase in spasticity is expected	• Check with CNS if any baclofen is lost during surgical procedure • Observe for any signs, and report to medical team • Oral anti-spasticity drug treatment may be commenced or increased to cover this period

Problem 4	Expected outcome	Nursing intervention
Risk of infection/haematoma at wound sites[4]	Any signs of infection/meningitis/ haematoma will be detected and treatment commenced promptly	Observe lumbar and abdomen wound sites for signs of: • Redness • Swelling • Tenderness 4-hourly temperatures until clips removed **Clip removal** Abdomen 7 days Date: _____ Lumbar 10 days (If catheter replaced) Date: _____ If patient is to be discharged before date of clip removal, organise for district nurse to remove clips and send home with clip remover
Problem 5	**Expected outcome**	**Nursing intervention**
Changes in level of spasticity throughout admission may affect PWS's ability to carry out activities or to be cared for	Accurate identification of any changes in function	• Identify any changes in level of function, and assist with care as required to promote safety • Liaise with spasticity and community teams
Problem 6	**Expected outcome**	**Nursing intervention**
(a) Person needs to feel prepared to go home with replacement pump implant in situ	PWS (or carer) demonstrates knowledge about the pump, its function and emergency situations	• CNS to give verbal and written information on pump system, side-effects, emergency contact procedure and alarm systems • Nurses to ensure PWS and/or carer can describe side-effects and what action they would take in an emergency • CNS to give PWS pump identification card • CNS to demonstrate alarm system to PWS and family • CNS to arrange follow-up in outpatient spasticity review and refill clinic • Nurses to ensure PWS and carer aware of review date
(b) Community team need to be aware of discharge and that a new intrathecal pump has been implanted	The community team state they have received enough information	• Medical team to contact GP • Nurses to contact district nurse • Nurses to ensure ward clerk sends information pack to GP and community teams at least 2 days before discharge

REFERENCES

1. Fox S, Krnjevic K, Morris ME, Puil E, Werman R. Action of baclofen on mammalian synaptic transmission. Neuroscience 1978;3:495–515.

2. Davies J. Selective depression of synaptic excitation in cat spinal neurones by baclofen: An iontophoretic study. Br J Pharmacol 1981;72:373–84.

3. Davidoff RA, Sears ES. The effects of Lioresal on synaptic activity in the isolated spinal cord. Neurology 1974;24:957–63.

4. Jarrett L, Leary SM, Porter B et al. Managing spasticity in people with multiple sclerosis. A goal orientated approach to intrathecal baclofen therapy. Int J MS Care 2001;3:2–11.

5. Lioresal Data Sheet. Lioresal©Intrathecal Baclofen Injection. Minneapolis: Medtronic, 1996.

6. Zierski J, Muller H, Dralle D, Wurdinger T. Implanted pump systems for treatment of spasticity. Acta Neurochir Suppl 1988;43:94–9.

7. Muller-Schwefe G, Penn RD. Physostigmine in the treatment of intrathecal baclofen overdose. J Neurosurg 1989;71:273–5.

8. Coffey RJ, Edgar TS, Franscisco GE et al. Abrupt withdrawal from intrathecal baclofen: recognition and management of a potentially life-threatening syndrome. Arch Phys Med Rehabil 2002;83:735–41.

9. Porter B. A review of intrathecal baclofen on the management of spasticity. Br J Nurs 1997;6:253–62.

Appendix 9

Specific competencies for intrathecal baclofen specialist nurses

The demonstration of intrathecal baclofen (ITB) nursing competencies includes presentation of evidence that illustrates learning about the subject and skill development. This evidence can come from various sources.	
A	Audit/data collection
O	Observation of practice
D	Documents: proposals, reports, strategies, standards, guidelines, policies, appraisals
L	Learning evidence: reflection, certificates, personal development plan, learning outcomes, study programmes

ITB Nurse Specialist	Evidence of achieving competence

Nurses' role in managing spasticity
 	
1. Demonstrate ability to be sensitive and supportive to people with spasticity (PWS) when dealing with their needs both in person and over the telephone.
 	
2. Teach nurses and carers the basic neurophysiological principles underlying spasticity and other features of the upper motor neurone syndrome.
 	
3. Teach a PWS, their carers, other nurses and other junior healthcare professionals (HCP) about trigger factors that can increase spasticity and effective management techniques.
 	
4. Discuss and be able to educate ward nurses and other HCPs about the treatments for spasticity and the nurses' role with:
 	
    • Stretching, hoisting and positioning
 	
    • Oral drugs
 	
    • Focal treatments
 	
    • Generalised treatments
 	
5. Be able to present on external courses to multidisciplinary audiences.	

ITB Nurse Specialist	Evidence of achieving competence
Spasticity assessment clinic 1. Within a multidisciplinary team, assess and appropriately select people suitable for ITB trial. 2. Complete without supervision the initial teaching with individuals who are recommended for ITB therapy by the spasticity team. 3. Post clinic, commence discharge planning process by liaising with relevant hospital and community teams.	
Arranging admissions 1. Continue with education of PWS by telephone without supervision. 2. Act as a key worker for the PWS throughout the admission, discharge and follow-up process. 3. Arrange all ITB admissions and liaise with appropriate hospital and community teams.	
ITB trial Carry out the following without supervision: 1. Continue spasticity assessment in the inpatient setting. 2. Complete spasticity measures with physiotherapist (PT). Demonstrate understanding of the significance of the measures and the importance of reviewing these measures after each trial. Monitor effect on PWS of being measured. 3. Together with the PWS and the team, agree on a goal of treatment. Demonstrate appropriate review of this goal after each trial. 4. Organise with the ward nurses the necessary equipment for the safe administration of the trial injection and to complete the observations following the injection. 5. Educate and support ward nursing team regarding trial process. 6. Educate and support medical team in carrying out ITB trial injection. 7. Evaluate effects of at least two trials with PWS and team using both subjective and objective information collected during the assessment and measures process. 8. Decide on future plan with multidisciplinary team and PWS.	
ITB implant Carry out the following without supervision: 1. Liaise with PWS regarding site for pump implant. 2. Continue education of PWS, reiterate implications (both positive and negative) of pump. 3. Liaise and coordinate with surgical team regarding equipment for implant and surgery time. 4. Attend theatre, ensuring that all equipment required is available and working. 5. Liaise with surgeon regarding site for implant, and record length of catheter removed during surgery. 6. With medical staff, calculate initial priming and starting dose. Programme pump while PWS is still in recovery.	

ITB Nurse Specialist	Evidence of achieving competence

7. Describe your role, identifying boundaries and when and where you would seek help within the different phases:
 	
    (a) Pre-operative
 	
    (b) Peri-operative
 	
    (c) Recovery phase
 	
    (d) Post-operative care on the ward
 	
    (e) Discharge planning
 	
Plan for discharge:
 	
8. Educate PWS and carer about pump alarm system and when it would be necessary to seek help.
 	
9. Educate community teams about ITB therapy, potential side-effects and procedure for getting help if problems occur.
 	
10. Prepare joint report with therapy teams.
 	
11. Arrange outpatient appointments to review spasticity and pump effectiveness.	

ITB pump replacement Carry out without supervision as for ITB implant, but in addition: 1. Monitor dates of potential replacements and prepare PWS for potential need for replacement. Liaise with community teams, carers and family members as appropriate. 2. Update PWS on any changes in the technology of the replacement pumps. 3. Educate PWS on potential changes in their degree of spasticity management during the replacement phase.	
Coordinating outpatient clinic Carry out the following without supervision: 1. Manage appointments according to reservoir refill dates. 2. Coordinate outpatient clinic and liaise with appropriate staff regarding transport, appointment times, etc. 3. Organise ITB prescriptions with pharmacy. 4. Organise emergency outpatient appointments if required. 5. Manage stocks of equipment: baclofen pumps, catheters, refill kits, 20 ml syringes, gauze, plasters, needles, etc. 6. Be able to effectively programme the pumps and maintain accurate records and printouts from the programmer. 7. Demonstrate competence at completing the pump refill procedure and effectively address pump problems and adverse events as they arise. 8. Educate new medical staff on all aspects of the ITB service, including how to use the programmer in both emergency and non-urgent situations. 9. Educate on-call medical teams as appropriate.	

ITB Nurse Specialist	Evidence of achieving competence
Managing the telephone helpline Carry out the following without supervision: 1. Manage the voice mail by regularly checking it and taking appropriate action with calls. 2. Demonstrate clear clinical reasoning and action when dealing with adverse events that may be related to pump or catheter malfunction. 3. Educate the ward nurses to manage the helpline out of hours and take appropriate action. 4. If necessary, organise urgent outpatient appointments or admissions when spasticity symptoms occur or alarms sound.	
Other 1. Manage stock levels of equipment and maintain accurate financial databases, ensuring that a clear financial audit trail for the service is available. 2. Ensure that database of equipment, i.e. serial numbers, product numbers and patient details, is accurate and up to date for use as a tracking system should equipment failure occur.	
Signature of Nurse　　　　　**Print name**	**Date**
Signature of Assessor　　　　**Print name**	**Date**
Signature of Manager　　　　**Print name**	**Date**

Appendix 10

Physiotherapy guidelines for intrathecal baclofen therapy

TRIAL OF INTRATHECAL BACLOFEN (ITB) THERAPY

The main responsibilities of the physiotherapist in conjunction with the clinical nurse specialist (CNS) are to:

- assess the individual's spasticity within 24 hours of admission
- record baseline outcome measures and agree the main goal of treatment with the individual
- repeat baseline measures with the CNS 4 hours after each trial injection
- attend ward rounds and give feedback from the physiotherapist's perspective
- prepare a joint therapy report with the CNS

PUMP IMPLANT

- If required, chest physiotherapy is carried out prior to surgery.
- Ensure that the individual is out of bed as soon as possible after surgery (at least 1 day post operation).
- Ensure that physiotherapy and wheelchair service follow-up is arranged in the community if required.
- Write a joint therapy report with the CNS.

PUMP REPLACEMENT

Individuals are likely to be admitted at short notice.

- Assess the individual's spasticity within 24 hours of admission.
- Record baseline outcome measures and agree the main goal of continuing treatment.
- Consider whether further physiotherapy input is required on discharge, and arrange if necessary.
- Consider if a wheelchair review is required.
- Write a joint therapy report with the CNS.

PUMP REFILL

The CNS and a doctor jointly run the refill clinic. The individual's spasticity management is reviewed, the intrathecal baclofen pumps are refilled and the prescription is reviewed. The physiotherapist's role is as follows:

1. Reassess and monitor individuals with new implantation of an intrathecal baclofen pump over the first year:
   - At the outpatient refill clinic, specifically reassess and measure tone, spasms, joint range, and goal achievement.
   - Review local therapy arrangements, seating and home exercise programme.

2. Be available on the clinic day to respond to requests by the clinic team for a physiotherapy assessment, and provide appropriate intervention as necessary.

3. Provide a yearly physiotherapy review for individuals on established ITB therapy, including assessment, outcome measures and review of therapy needs, and provide intervention as appropriate. Provide feedback to the team. Assessments can be pre-arranged before the time in clinic so that this does not impact on the clinic length and to allow full assessment and feedback.

Appendix 11

Surgical procedure for intrathecal baclofen pump placement

- The patient is anaesthetised and placed, flexed, in the lateral position, with the upper arm elevated on an arm support – thus exposing the abdomen for the pump placement, but also ensuring the true upright position, easing the insertion of the lumbar catheter.

- A horizontal incision over the lumbar 3/4 space of 4–5 cm has proved better than a longitudinal incision, which has been abandoned as it restricts catheter anchorage.

- The Touhy needle is inserted just off the midline to pass through the erector spinae muscle rather than through the interspinous ligament. This reduces cerebral spinal fluid (CSF) tracking back, perhaps because the muscle makes a more permanent seal.

- The needle is passed directly through to the CSF rather than using the standard air-injection method. Once the dura has been penetrated and clear CSF flow demonstrated, the stylet of the needle is replaced to minimise leakage.

- The catheter with guidewire is inserted cephalad to about 10 cm or between the 3rd and 4th marks. If it will not initially pass, the needle is withdrawn a few millimetres, which usually unblocks the tip opening, although CSF flow must be reconfirmed. The needle and then the guidewire are removed, the latter by holding the catheter at the entry point to the spine and pulling the guidewire at the loose end. The catheter is best anchored using a curved

channel, as this takes strain off the entry point and directs the catheter towards the pump.

- The abdominal pocket in the lower-abdominal quadrant is fashioned at the same time by a second surgeon. An oblique 10–12 cm *straight* incision is sufficient. This avoids a relatively avascular curved flap and an incision line that lies over the pump itself, both of which can predispose to infection. The pocket is then fashioned medial to this incision; a dummy pump is useful to check the size required. The sleeve is not employed routinely as it may cause difficulties during pump replacement. However, in an obese patient, it is advisable to locate the pump on the abdominal fascia (to avoid migration and rotation), using the eyes on the pump body and a stout non-absorbable suture. This does not seem to be necessary in slim patients.

- As the first surgeon is inevitably still at work creating the anchorage for the catheter, the pocket can be packed with a betadine-soaked swab to both minimise oozing and reduce infection.

- Any tunnelling device can connect the two incisions, and once the pump has been prepared, it can be connected to the suitably shortened catheter, leaving enough slack to allow some movement with subsequent spasms. The pump is inserted with the catheter lying behind it, and the incisions are closed.

Appendix 12

Refill procedure for Medtronic electronic pumps

PREPARATION

The refill procedure involves a specific set of tasks that must be followed precisely to ensure the individual's safety. It is imperative that aseptic technique be followed throughout the procedure in order to maintain sterility of the pump reservoir, fluid pathway and device pocket.

OBTAINING EQUIPMENT AND MEDICATION

The equipment required for refill of the Medtronic SynchroMed system is as follows:

- intrathecal baclofen
- Medtronic refill kit (Figure 1)

Figure 1

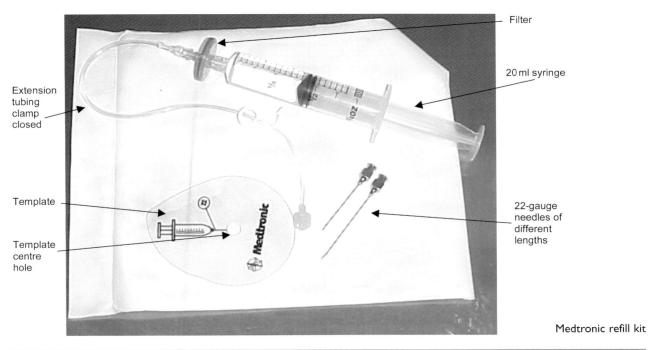

Filter

Extension tubing clamp closed

Template

Template centre hole

20 ml syringe

22-gauge needles of different lengths

Medtronic refill kit

- programmer
- 20 ml syringe
- 21-gauge needle
- swabs
- skin-preparation fluid
- sterile gloves
- small dressing/plaster

THE REFILL PROCEDURE

- Assemble the components listed above.
- Identify the pump model, the reservoir size, and the locations of the centre reservoir fill port and side catheter access port.
- Perform telemetry to check current pump status and determine the expected volume of fluid remaining in the pump reservoir.
- Open the refill kit and ensure that all the pieces are connected securely together (they can become loose in transit, which can risk allowing air to get in the system and the pump becoming overpressurised).
- Prepare the injection site by cleansing with a quick-drying skin-cleansing agent (e.g. Betadine).
- Using a sterile procedure, draw up the baclofen via a 21-gauge needle into a luer lock 20 ml syringe (draw up the required amount depending on the size of pump reservoir).

- Remove the needle and discard safely. Attach the filter and prime it. Leave on the sterile field.
- Assemble the 22-gauge Huber-type needle and extension tubing set with the clamp in the closed position.
- Palpate the pump and hold onto two sides. Place the template over the pump, aligning its edges with those of the pump. If the pump has a side catheter access port, locate it so that you can avoid accessing it in the next step. The catheter access port leads directly to the catheter and hence the intrathecal space – it would be extremely dangerous to inject baclofen directly through this port, especially the volume needed for a refill.
- Insert the needle through the template centre hole (Figure 2) and into the pump septum and drug reservoir until the needle touches the needle stop (excessive force could damage the needle tip and possibly the septum when removed).
- Attach an empty 20 ml syringe to the end of the extension tubing, release the clamp and withdraw the fluid from the reservoir using gentle negative pressure. Empty the reservoir completely until air bubbles are present in the extension tube.
- Check the amount withdrawn: it should be approximately equal to the previously noted reservoir volume from the pump status screen.
- Close the clamp and remove the 20 ml syringe, leaving the needle and tubing in situ. (Note:

Figure 2

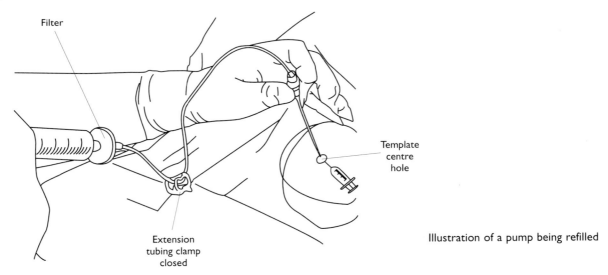

Filter

Template centre hole

Extension tubing clamp closed

Illustration of a pump being refilled

Failure to close the clamp completely could result in pump contamination or overpressurisation of the pump reservoir if air entered.)

- Attach the drug-filled syringe with filter to the extension tubing. Release the clamp, slowly injecting at an infusion rate not greater than 1 ml every 3 seconds. (Note: Do not force the injection, as this can activate a safety valve, which can prevent the refill from occurring.)
- When filling is complete, maintain slight, positive pressure on the syringe.
- Remove the needle and syringe and discard safely.
- Remove the cleaning agent from the individual's skin and apply a plaster if required.
- Programme the appropriate parameters (note that the reservoir volume will always need to be amended after a refill) and perform telemetry to update the pump.
- Produce two print-outs of the dose: one for the nursing and one for the medical notes. Some individuals also like to have a copy. The doctor and nurse check that the readout is correct before the individual leaves the clinic.
- Note the low-reservoir alarm date and organise the next refill visit before this date.

KEY SAFETY ISSUES

- Injection of the drug during the refill procedure must be through the centre reservoir fill port. Improper injection through the side catheter access port or into the pump pocket may result in a clinically significant or fatal drug overdose. Always identify the locations of the centre reservoir fill port and side catheter access port. The needles in the refill kit should not pass through these unless excessively forced. It is imperative that the needles, templates and other accessories provided with the Medtronic refill kit be used to prevent this from occurring. A dedicated catheter access port kit is available if a radiopaque dye study needs to be carried out.
- Failure to empty the reservoir prior to refilling could lead to overfilling of the reservoir, which may lead to overpressurisation and damage to the pump mechanism.
- If the position of the pump cannot be established, an X-ray can help to determine the pump position and the reservoir access point. Pumps occasionally have been reported as turning over, preventing access to the reservoir.

Appendix 13

How intrathecal phenol may help you manage your lower-limb spasticity

Intrathecal phenol

Phenol is a drug that if expertly injected into your spine damages motor nerves and relieves persistent spasticity, spasms and pain in your legs. This can make your legs easier to position and more comfortable when you are sitting or lying down.

Potential outcomes

The potential outcomes are to reduce:

- spasticity – often described as a feeling of stiffness in your legs
- spasms – or involuntary contractions of muscles – which can make your legs suddenly move towards or away from your body
- pain in your legs

Minimising these symptoms can have an impact on the way you can be positioned in your bed and chair. It can make you feel more comfortable and ease the effort of washing and dressing your lower half.

Assessment and measurement

The initial treatment requires an inpatient hospital stay. During the first 2 days, a doctor, a nurse and a physiotherapist, all of whom specialise in managing spasticity, will assess you.

The assessments will identify the main problems that your spasticity and spasms cause you on a daily basis. In addition, the specialist nurse and physiotherapist will want to move and stretch your legs so that they can gain a better understanding of how your legs feel when moved. They will also measure the position your legs are in when you are sitting and lying. If you have pain when being moved, you will only be moved within the limits of your pain – in other words, you will guide how much your legs are moved.

The assessment and measures enable the team to give you clear guidance on how they think the intrathecal phenol may help you. Together with the team, you will identify a goal amenable to treatment with intrathecal phenol that would have an impact on your daily life.

Throughout this process, the spasticity management team will discuss all the information with you and, if you wish, your family. The decision as to whether intrathecal phenol is the right treatment for you can then be made together.

Injection process

There are two distinct stages to the treatment:

1. A trial injection of anaesthetic
2. The phenol injection(s)

Each injection targets one leg, so if you have spasticity in both of your legs you will need two phenol injections – one to target each leg. The most effective way to target the whole leg is to inject the drugs into your spine. Both the trial anaesthetic and phenol are injected into the liquid-filled cavity surrounding the spinal cord called the intrathecal space.

The trial injection

Firstly, we would give you a test injection of anaesthetic which allows you to experience the likely effect of the phenol injection with an anaesthetic drug that has a temporary effect (30 minutes to 2 hours). The injection is given via a lumbar puncture (which you may have had before), but instead of taking fluid from around the spinal cord, a small amount of drug is injected.

You will be asked to lie on your side; if this is difficult, do not worry, there will be equipment and team members to help you get into position and to support you.

Once you are lying on your side, a small area on your lower back will be made temporarily numb with local anaesthetic and then the test anaesthetic will be injected via a lumbar puncture into your spine. There should be little or no pain during the procedure.

Following the injection, you may need to be repositioned and tilted slightly forward to ensure that the drug reaches the right area in your spine. Your blood pressure and pulse will be recorded very regularly during this time.

You will need to stay in this position for 5 minutes after the trial injection. You will be supported to do this and a nurse will be with you at all times. After the time for the injection to work has elapsed, the nurse specialist and physiotherapist will reassess the effect on your legs with you. A family member or carer can be present for this assessment if you wish. The temporary effect can last between 30 minutes and 2 hours, or sometimes longer. This period is the main decision-making time, as you will now have had all the information and be experiencing what the effect of the injection feels like. Most people find it useful to have a significant other with them at this time, so you can discuss the outcome and decide whether it would be beneficial to you.

After returning to the ward, your blood pressure, pulse and temperature will be recorded for a short time. You will be able to eat and drink and if possible sit out of bed.

The intrathecal phenol injections

The procedure is the same as described above for the trial injection, although the drug injected is phenol and you will need to maintain the position that you are put in after the injection for 20 minutes. This can be a bit uncomfortable, but we will do everything we can to support you and there will be a nurse with you throughout this time.

Potential side-effects during or immediately after the treatment

- There is a possibility that your blood pressure could drop, which could make you feel slightly light-headed or nauseous. If this occurs, it tends to do so just after the injection and is usually short-lived; the doctor and nurse will closely monitor you during this time.
- A headache may occur afterward, but should last no longer than a few days.

Longer-lasting potential side-effects

- The injections may cause your legs to feel numb. For some people, this different sensation can take time to get used to. The numbness may increase the risk of pressure sores, as it may prevent you from noticing an area that would previously have been uncomfortable or painful. It is important that someone is able to monitor your skin for any signs of redness or breakdown on a very regular basis. In addition, you may not be able to feel when someone touches your legs or lower body.
- Your legs may feel very weak, but you should not feel weak above the waist.
- Intrathecal phenol may interfere with bladder or bowel control. If this occurs, it tends to be temporary (4–5 weeks), but could have a longer-term effect. If these functions are already affected (for example if you use an indwelling catheter or regularly use suppositories or enemas), the injection is unlikely to cause any extra problems. Options to manage your bladder and bowels in both the short- and long-term following the intrathecal phenol will be discussed with you.

Community nursing teams often have expertise in supporting people to manage their bladder and bowels; it may be helpful to involve them in the discussions.

- The injections can affect your sexual function. For men, it can reduce the effectiveness of erections, while for women the reduction in lower-half sensation may minimise what they feel.

A team member will discuss these side-effects with you before the doctor asks you to consent to going ahead with the treatment.

Discharge

You are normally able to go home the day after the last phenol injection.

Ongoing treatment

In total, it is common for people to require three injections: a trial injection and two phenol injections (one to target each leg). The effects of intrathecal phenol can be permanent and there is no method of reversing the procedure, but sometimes the effect wears off over time. If the spasticity, spasms or pain return, there should be no problem about doing the procedure again. Normally, this is done as a day case. You can re-access the service by either you or a member of your family or community team contacting the specialist nurse for spasticity management.

The specialist nurse for spasticity management or the pain management nurses can be contacted on the telephone numbers below if you have any further questions or concerns:

Telephone numbers

_____

_____

_____

Appendix 14

Nursing care plan for intrathecal phenol therapy

Problem 1	Expected outcome	Nursing intervention
The person with spasticity (PWS) requires information and education to make informed decisions about proceeding with the trial of intrathecal phenol (IP) therapy IP is administered for the treatment of severe lower-limb spasticity and associated pain. Phenol is a neurolytic agent that causes axonal degeneration and indiscriminate destruction of motor and sensory nerves. When mixed with glycerol, it diffuses from the solution into cerebrospinal fluid (CSF) and nerve tissue Anaesthetic agents such as bupivacaine work by temporarily blocking nerve transmission by decreasing sodium channel permeability. Bupivacaine is administered during the trial phase to enable the PWS to experience what may be achieved by phenol injection and for the team to assess whether the goal can be achieved and the extent of any contractures	PWS makes an informed decision	• Liaise with spasticity nurse specialist (CNS) • CNS to educate/inform PWS about IP, the injection process and its potential effects and side-effects with a member of ward nursing staff present • Ward nurses reinforce information as necessary and continue teaching Education/information should include: **A description of the procedure:** This is a specialised injection and requires an expert medical injector. It involves a spinal needle being inserted into the intrathecal space at a lumbar spine level to specifically target the person's lower-limb spasticity. This level is determined by an assessment carried out by the spasticity team **The care immediately required after the injection:** CNS will monitor the person until the block has fixed and their observations are stable

Problem 2	Expected outcome	Nursing intervention
(a) PWS needs to have a spasticity assessment and baseline measures recorded pre injection	Accurate record of spasticity and spasms to ascertain efficacy of treatment	• CNS and physiotherapist (PT) will complete an assessment and measures pre and post injections • Nurses to give feedback on how spasticity affects nursing care
(b) The main problem and goal of treatment need to be established	Agreed goal: _____ _____	• Medical team, CNS and PT will discuss and agree goal with PWS
(c) Changes in level of spasticity throughout admission may affect PWS's ability to carry out activities or to be cared for	Accurate identification of any changes in function	• Identify any changes in level of function or care required • Liaise with spasticity management team
(d) Trial of anaesthetic attempts to assess if IP will improve current spasticity management of PWS. Therefore the current spasticity management strategies need to continue	PWS will continue their regular spasticity management strategies	• Continue with normal spasticity management, i.e. oral drug regime, stretching programme, effective management of bladder and bowels • **PWS will continue to take their normal oral drugs unless indicated by the medical team throughout the trial period. If side-effects occur, contact the medical team**
Problem 3	Expected outcome	Nursing intervention
(a) PWS needs to be prepared for procedure (trial anaesthetic or phenol)	PWS is ready for the procedure	• Complete pre-procedure checklist • Nurses to familiarise themselves with level of spasticity (stiffness felt in limbs), frequency and intensity of spasms prior to treatment to enable assessment of changes post injection • Record neurological observations, blood pressure (BP), pulse, respiration (resp.) rate and oxygen saturations pre treatment • PWS will be nil-by-mouth for 4 hours prior to procedure. Continue with prescribed medication unless instructed otherwise • Pain management team to be informed if PWS is receiving anticoagulant therapy or non-steroidal anti-inflammatory medication
(b) Anti-emboli stockings are rarely required for people having IP therapy	To prevent skin breakdown	• Often in people with severe spasticity and spasms, anti-emboli stockings are difficult to apply and keep in a position that will promote skin integrity. Passive limb exercises are the preferred method of preventing deep-vein thrombosis (DVT)

Problem 4	Expected outcome	Nursing intervention
(a) PWS is monitored for potential side-effects, including hypotension, infection, CSF leakage, respiratory depression and low-pressure headache	Side-effects are detected early and prompt action taken	• BP, pulse, resp. rate and pulse oximetry are monitored every 30 minutes for 2 hours on return to ward. If stable, they may then be discontinued • Temperature should be monitored daily until discharge and 4-hourly if elevated • Check the lumbar puncture site to ensure no signs of infection or CSF leakage • Signs of low-pressure headache need to be monitored for. Classically, this presents as a severe headache when the person sits up that is relieved when they lie down
(b) Effects of phenol are assessed and remeasured	To assess effect of injections	• CNS and PT repeat measures to assess effect of injection and whether the goal is achieved • Nursing staff feedback changes in care requirements
Problem 5	**Expected outcome**	**Nursing intervention**
(a) PWS is prepared for discharge and is aware of potential complications: • Reduced bladder/bowel function • Reduced perineal and lower-limb sensation • Reduced sexual function • Lower-limb weakness • Potential of DVT	PWS is aware of potential side-effects, contact details and follow-up arrangements	• CNS to discuss side-effects with PWS and carer. Ward nursing staff to support CNS • CNS to provide follow-up details and contact information
(b) PWS's community team are aware of procedure	PWS has community support when discharged	• Medical team write discharge report • Ward staff to update district nursing team on all nursing care needs • CNS and PT write joint nursing/therapy report, which is sent to relevant community team members

CHECKLIST FOR INDIVIDUALS HAVING INTRATHECAL PHENOL

(To be completed by ward nurse prior to each procedure. Please indicate 'Yes' or 'No' in the boxes unless otherwise stated)

Name:	Hospital No.:		DOB:		
Ward:		**Bupivacaine Date:**	**Phenol 1 Date:**	**Phenol 2 Date:**	
Baseline obs: BP, TPR recorded prior to each injection					
Name band correct and in situ					
Cannula/IV fluids in situ					
Consent form completed					
Target side (right or left)					
NBM from (indicate time in box)					
Blood results in medical notes (Bloods to be checked by doctor prior to first injection)			✕	✕	
Is the person prescribed anticoagulants or NSAIDs					

Pre injection

- Nursing staff should complete a pre-operative checklist (see above), a baseline recording of temperature, blood pressure, respiration and pulse rate prior to the intrathecal anaesthetic trial and the phenol injections.
- The individual should be nil-by-mouth for 4 hours prior to the injections, but may take medication with a sip of water.
- The injector should be informed if the individual is taking anticoagulant therapy or non-steroidal anti-inflammatory drugs (NSAIDs).

Post injection

The main risks following intrathecal local anaesthetic or phenol are hypotension, infection, cerebrospinal fluid (CSF) leak and unwanted effects of extension of block (e.g. respiratory depression).

- A specialist nurse will supervise the individual immediately following the injection until it has been established that the block is fixed and the blood pressure, pulse and respiration rate are within an acceptable range for that individual.
- Once the individual returns to the ward, the nurses will continue to measure temperature, blood pressure, pulse and respiration rate every 30 minutes for 2 hours; then, if stable, the observations can be discontinued. The temperature should continue to be monitored at least once a day prior to discharge. However, if the temperature is raised above the individual's baseline then recordings should be carried out 4-hourly.
- The nurses will assess the individual for signs of a low-pressure headache, i.e. occipital headache (worse when sitting up), and manage according to medical advice.
- The nurses will also observe the puncture site for leakage of CSF, and manage according to medical advice.

Index

Page numbers in italics refer to tables and figures.